The Book of
Exercise and Yoga
for Those with Multiple Sclerosis

A Program to Improve Balance and
Manage Symptoms of Pain and Fatigue
2nd Edition

ISBN number: 978-1466417687

Published by:
Living Well Yoga and Fitness
PO Box 1057
Montauk, NY 11954
(631) 259-1385
www.lwyf.org

Acknowledgments

My sincere gratitude to my students living with Multiple Sclerosis who face each day's challenges with humor, grace and courage. You are, and will continue to be, an inspiration to us all.

Dedication

This book is dedicated to those living with Multiple Sclerosis and their families. Proceeds from the sale of this book will be donated to help find a cure.

Preface
Using Movement and Meditation to Manage
the Symptoms of Multiple Sclerosis

"Nothing in life is to be feared. It is only to be understood."
- Marie Curie

What Is Multiple Sclerosis

Multiple sclerosis (MS) is a serious chronic and progressive illness that affects the body's nervous system. It attacks the brain and spinal cord resulting in sensations such as numbness, loss of muscle control, vision, balance, and/or thinking ability. MS is an autoimmune disease. Autoimmune diseases are those whereby the body's immune system, which normally targets and destroys substances foreign to the body (such as bacteria), mistakenly attacks normal tissues. With MS, the immune system attacks the central nervous system and damages the nerves of the brain and spinal cord.

The central nervous system consists of the brain, spinal cord and nerves that act as the body's messenger system. The nerves are covered by a fatty substance called myelin. Myelin insulates the nerves and aids in the transmission of nerve impulses, or messages between the brain and other parts of the body. These nerve impulses control muscle movements, such as walking and talking. Multiple Sclerosis causes a buildup of scar tissue (sclerosis) in the brain and spinal cord, and myelin can be lost in multiple areas. These damaged areas are also known as plaques or lesions. The scar tissue or plaques form when the myelin that covers the nerves is destroyed, (demyelination). Sometimes the nerve fiber itself can be damaged. Without the myelin covering, electrical signals transmitted throughout the brain and spinal cord are disrupted or halted. The brain then becomes unable to send and receive messages. When this breakdown of communication occurs the symptoms of MS appear. The type and severity of symptoms, and the course of MS varies widely, partly due to the location of the scar tissue and the extent of demyelination.

Types of Multiple Sclerosis
People with MS may have one of four courses of disease, each of which is identified by the types of exacerbations or relapses that occur and all forms can be be mild, moderate, or severe.

Exacerbation.
An exacerbation (also known as an attack, relapse, or a flare) is a sudden worsening of symptoms, or the appearance of new symptoms, which lasts at least 24 hours and is separated from a previous exacerbation by at least one month, with no progression of the disease between attacks. An exacerbation may be mild or severe enough to interfere with daily activities. An exacerbation of MS can last days to weeks and is caused by an area of

inflammation in the central nervous system. This is followed by the destruction of myelin.

Pseudoexacerbations are situations that temporarily aggravate MS problems. Sometimes an increase in symptoms has nothing to do with the underlying MS, but is caused by factors such as fever, infection, or hot weather that can temporarily aggravate MS problems. For example some people experience a worsening of symptoms during or after periods of intense stress.

Remission.

A remission does not mean that all the symptoms of MS disappear, but rather that a person with MS returns to the baseline that existed before the last exacerbation began.

1. Relapsing-Remitting MS

This type of MS is characterized by unpredictable exacerbations with a worsening of neurologic function and symptoms. This is followed by full, partial, or no recovery of some function. These attacks may evolve over several days to weeks and recovery can take weeks and sometimes months.

2. Primary-Progressive MS

This type of MS is characterized by a slow but nearly continuous worsening of the disease from onset, with no distinct relapses or remissions. However, there are variations in rates of progression over time and there may be temporary minor improvements. This form is relatively rare, occurring in just 15 percent of all people with MS, but it is the most common type of MS in people who develop the disease after the age of 40.

3. Secondary-Progressive MS

People with this type of MS experience an initial period of relapsing-remitting disease, followed by a steadily worsening disease course with or without occasional flare-ups, or remissions. The progressive part of the disease may begin shortly after the onset of MS, or it may occur years or decades later.

4. Progressive-Relapsing MS

In this type of MS people experience a steady worsening disease from the onset but also have clear acute relapses or exacerbations with or without recovery. In contrast to relapsing-remitting MS, the periods between relapses are characterized by continuing disease progression. This type is relatively rare affecting approximately five percent of all cases.

Causes of Multiple Sclerosis

While the exact cause of MS is unknown, most researchers believe that the damage to myelin results from an abnormal response by the body's immune system. Scientists do not yet know what triggers the immune system to do this, however several factors may be involved such as:

> Genetics

Researchers believe that MS may be inherited. First, second, and third degree relatives of people with MS are at increased risk of developing the disease. Siblings of an affected person have a two to five percent risk of developing MS. Researchers believe that there is more than one gene that makes a person more likely to get MS. Some scientists theorize that MS develops because a person is born with a genetic predisposition to react to some environmental agent, which upon exposure triggers an autoimmune response.

> Environmental triggers.

Different populations and ethnic groups have a markedly different prevalence of MS. The disease is especially common in Scotland, Scandinavia, and throughout northern Europe. In the U.S. the prevalence of MS is higher in whites than in other racial groups. Also, MS is a disease of temperate climates. In both hemispheres, its prevalence increases with distance from the equator.

> Viruses

Some studies have suggested that viruses such as measles, herpes, and the flu may be associated with MS. To date, however, this belief has not been proven.

> Hormones

There is growing evidence suggesting that hormones, including sex hormones can affect the immune system. For example, both estrogen and progesterone (two important female sex hormones) and testosterone (the primary male hormone) may suppress some immune activity.

Diagnosis of Multiple Sclerosis

At this time, no single test is available to identify or rule out MS. Several tests and procedures are needed. These include:

> A complete medical history that examines the overall view of the individual's health picture, including symptoms and when they began.

> Nervous system functioning. Testing of reflexes, balance, coordination, and vision as well as checking for areas of numbness.

> Diagnostic Tests such as:
- Magnetic Resonance Imaging (MRI) scan which gives a detailed view of the brain. This scan makes it possible to visualize and count white matter lesions (damaged areas or scars) in the brain and spinal cord.
- Evoked potential tests, which measure how quickly and accurately a person's nervous system responds to certain stimulation.
- A spinal tap, which checks spinal fluid for signs of the disease.

- Examination of the cerebrospinal fluid. This fluid found in the central nervous system can provide clues to the diagnosis of MS and other diseases.

There are two basic signs that are required to confirm the diagnosis of MS:
1. Signs of the disease in different parts of the nervous system.
2. Signs of at least two separate relapses or exacerbations of the disease.

Who gets Multiple Sclerosis

According to the National Multiple Sclerosis Society, MS affects approximately 400,000 Americans, and every week about 200 people are diagnosed. Worldwide, MS may affect 2.5 million individuals. It is a frequent cause of neurological disability beginning in early to middle adulthood.

MS FACTS
- Most people with MS are diagnosed between the ages of 20 and 50 and its occurrence is unusual before adolescence. A person has an increased risk of developing the disease from the teen years to age 50, with the risk gradually declining thereafter.
- MS is two to three times more common in females then males.
- Studies indicate that genetic factors make certain individuals more susceptible than others.
- MS occurs more commonly among people with northern European ancestry, but people of African, Asian, and Hispanic backgrounds are not immune.
- MS is not contagious.
- There is no cure for MS yet, but there are FDA-approved medications that have been shown to modify or slow down the underlying course of MS. Advances in treating and understanding MS are made every year and progress in research to find a cure is very encouraging.
- MS was among the first diseases to be described scientifically. The 19th-century doctors did not understand what they saw and recorded, but medical drawings done as early as 1838 clearly show what we today recognize as MS.
- MS is not usually fatal. Most people with MS have a near normal life span. Most deaths associated with MS are due to complications in advanced, progressive stages of the disease. Effective early treatment of MS should help to prevent those complications.
- The majority of people with MS do not become severely disabled. Many people with MS remain able to walk without help. However, the likelihood of needing a mobility device increases the longer someone has MS. In addition, people who are still able to walk may use a wheelchair, cane, scooter, or other device to conserve energy or prevent injury from falls.
- MS does not always prevent people from working. There is no scientific evidence that the normal stress of working has any effect on MS. But symptoms such as fatigue, can cause problems on the job. Approximately 30 percent of people with MS are working full-time after 20 years.

➤ Most women with MS find their symptoms lessen during pregnancy. Then, the risk of an attack rises somewhat in the first six months after delivery. Overall, pregnancy and childbirth have no long-term effect on MS. Those who worry that their children will develop MS should know that the risk is actually very small: somewhere between one and five percent.

➤ Intimacy does not have to disappear from the lives of couples when one partner has MS. Instead, partners can find approaches that overcome the barriers.

Symptoms of Multiple Sclerosis

Multiple sclerosis symptoms generally appear between the ages of 20 and 40 and the onset may be dramatic, or so mild that a person doesn't even notice any symptoms until far later in the course of the disease. Multiple sclerosis follows a varied and unpredictable course. In many people, the disease starts with a single symptom, followed by months or even years without any progression of symptoms. In others, the symptoms become worse within weeks or months. It is important to understand that although a wide range of symptoms can occur, a given individual may experience only some of the symptoms and never have others. Some symptoms may occur once, resolve, and never return. Because MS is such an individual disease, it is not helpful to compare yourself with other people who have MS.

Some common symptoms of MS include:

✔ Fatigue. This is the most common symptom of MS. It is typically present in the mid afternoon and may consist of increased muscle weakness, mental fatigue, sleepiness, or drowsiness. As many as 75 to 95 percent of all people with MS have fatigue and 50 to 60 percent say that it's one of their worst problems. In fact, fatigue is one of the major reasons for unemployment among people with MS.

➤ Tingling, numbness, or other abnormal sensations. Many people with MS experience abnormal sensations such as "pins and needles," itching, burning, stabbing or tearing pains.

➤ Dizziness and loss of balance. Many people with MS complain of feeling "off balance" or lightheaded. Occasionally they may experience the feeling that they or their surroundings are spinning (vertigo). These symptoms occur due to damage to the nerve pathways that coordinate vision and other inputs into the brain needed to maintain balance.

➤ Weakness in one or more limbs.

➤ Blurred or double vision. Vision problems are relatively common in people with MS however most vision problems do not lead to blindness.

➤ Heat sensitivity. This is the appearance or worsening of symptoms when exposed to heat. This symptom occurs in most people with MS.

- Spasticity. Muscle spasms are a common and often debilitating symptom of MS and they usually affect the muscles of the legs and arms, and may interfere with a persons ability to move those muscles freely.

- Impaired thinking. Problems with thinking occur in about half of people with MS. For most, this means slowed thinking, decreased concentration, or decreased memory.

- Speech and swallowing problems. People with MS often have swallowing difficulties and speech problems.

- Tremors are fairly common in people with MS.

- Difficulty walking or lack of coordination is another very common symptom of MS. This problem can be related to muscle weakness and/or spasticity, but having balance problems or numbness in your feet can also make walking difficult.

- Depression is a common problem among people with MS.

Prognosis of Multiple Sclerosis

In general it is very difficult to predict the course of MS since it varies for each person. A diagnosis is based on the combination of problems, patterns of recurrence, which systems are impaired and your test results. There is no way to predict how each person's condition will progress. It often takes years before a doctor can be certain of an MS diagnosis and have some idea on how the disease will progress, but most people with MS can expect to live 95 percent of the normal life expectancy.

Treatments for Multiple Sclerosis

Prescription Drugs

There are several medications that may help manage the symptoms of MS. The helpful webpages section in the back of this book lists organizations that can provide information on current medications. However, most prescription drugs have possible side effects, and some drugs shouldn't be mixed with others. Before you start any prescription drug, make sure your doctor has a current list of all other medications you are taking including vitamins, minerals, and herbal or dietary products. Always ask your doctor about possible side effects and what to do if they occur. It's a good idea to get this information in writing and share it with family members and caregivers.

Diet

Healthy eating is important for everyone, but it is particularly important if you have a chronic illness, such as multiple sclerosis. Good nutrition, especially adequate calories and protein, helps maintain your body's store of protein, provides you with energy, and gives you a nutritional base to heal wounds and fight infection.

Some basic nutrition guidelines are:
- Eat a variety of foods from each food group.
- Maintain your weight through a proper balance of exercise and food.
- Choose foods low in saturated fat and cholesterol, unless otherwise directed by your healthcare provider.
- Limit sugar.
- Moderate your use of salt.
- If you choose to drink alcoholic beverages, do not consume more than one or two beverages per day. (Always consult with your doctor about alcohol consumption).
- Drink six to eight 8-ounce glasses of water per day.
- Limit caffeine consumption.

Exercise

Regular, moderate physical exercise is good for the body, mind, and spirit. For those with MS, exercise is an important tool to help maintain function, mobility, and help manage symptoms such as depression, fatigue, and weakness. Regular exercise can improve a loss of fitness caused by a sedentary lifestyle and be therapeutic for such MS-related problems as spasticity and poor balance. Exercise also builds a reserve of muscle strength and cardiovascular function. Then, if an attack or exacerbation of MS calls for a time-out from physical activity, the reserve is available. When the symptoms subside and you are able to go back to a more normal life, there is a better foundation on which to rebuild.

However, all benefits of exercise are short-term; that is, they fade away if exercise is discontinued. On the other hand, all exercise provides benefits. If you find you can't do what you used to do, don't give up. You can always modify or turn to something more feasible. Physical therapists and exercise physiologists can provide expert help. Exercise can help ease the symptoms of MS, but it's important to take certain precautions if you want your exercise program to be successful.

In the chapters that follow different types of exercise will be outlined as well as explanations of how they can help those with MS. It is important to take the suggestions as a guide only, and listen to your own body to determine what is right for you.

Note:

This book is provided as a helpful reference source only. It is not intended as a medical guide, or a guide for self-treatment. The suggestions herein are not intended to replace appropriate medical care. If you are concerned about your health or diagnosis, seek competent medical attention. This book offers techniques that may be helpful for those with Multiple Sclerosis. If you are living with another medical condition some of the suggestions in this book may be contraindicated for your condition. Check with your healthcare provider about the appropriateness of this program given your particular diagnosis.

Never exercise to the point of pain or strain, and discontinue exercising immediately if you experience pain or pressure in the chest, dizziness, nausea, extreme muscle soreness, or a worsening of symptoms. If you should experience any of the above, consult your health care provider immediately.

Table of Contents

Introduction

Making Exercise a Part of Your Day

"Life is not easy for any of us. But what of that? We must have perseverance
and above all confidence in ourselves. We must believe that we are gifted for
something and that this thing must be attained."
- Marie Curie

The benefits of regular exercise have been well documented. Hardly a day goes by when we are not reminded of its importance through news broadcasts, newspapers, and magazine articles. Regular exercise combined with other healthy lifestyle choices can help you manage weight, reduce blood pressure, cholesterol levels, and stress. It can also aid in the prevention and management of such conditions as diabetes, heart disease, cancer, arthritis, and MS. While exercise can help to moderate many conditions, it is especially crucial for those who are living with a chronic disease. In the case of Multiple Sclerosis (MS), the body is being affected by a progressive condition that can cause a loss of mobility. The ability to do everyday activities becomes more challenging as joints lose range of motion, muscles become weaker, balance is compromised, and fatigue worsens.

Activities of daily living, often called ADLs, include eating, dressing, bathing, sleeping, toileting, walking or moving about in general. Having Multiple Sclerosis can affect each of these. Some symptoms of MS (fatigue, slow movement, and balance problems) may worsen over time, and can make it more difficult to do such things as getting in and out of a car, standing up from a chair, or walking.

Addressing these symptoms with regular exercise may help to slow the progression of the disease as one maintains or even gains more mobility. An exercise program should consist of aerobic or cardiovascular exercise, strength training exercise, and stretching exercises. Regular aerobic exercise helps make the heart stronger and helps to increase lung capacity. Strength training exercises help to increase muscular strength. Stretching exercises help maintain joint range of motion. Each of the following chapters will explore different types of movement and discuss in detail how they can help.

Fitting exercise into your daily routine can be challenging especially when you are also dealing with a chronic disease. There are some steps you can take to make this easier:

1) Schedule your exercise session into your day as you would a doctor's appointment or a meeting with a friend, and do not break your appointment unless it is absolutely necessary. Postponing your designated time can become a habit too easy to maintain. This could result in neglecting exercise altogether. Exercise is an important component to your overall health. Your exercise schedule should be given a priority as important as a medical appointment.

2) Schedule your exercise routine for a time of day that works best for you. For those with MS, this means finding a time when have energy and feel your strongest. If you

know that you tend to get tired by late afternoon, make sure you schedule your session earlier in the day.

3) Exercising with a partner or friend is more enjoyable then going at it alone. It keeps you motivated and on track. Making an agreement to do this is a great way to help you stick to your routine. Even if you do not feel like exercising you may not want to let your partner down.

4) If you only have the time or energy to do just part of your usual routine, do what you can. Do not skip your exercise session just because you can only do part of it. Because unavoidable situations may occur to disrupt your routine, you may be tempted to skip it, a practice that too easily leads to breaking your exercise habit altogether. Missing one exercise session may tempt you to miss the next day, and before long you may stop exercising altogether. By doing what you can in the time allowed helps you to maintain a rhythm of regular exercise.

5) Should you fall off track, do not be too hard on yourself. Everyone experiences periods of slipping back into old habits and routines. The important thing is that you recognize this pattern and return quickly to healthier habits and lifestyle choices. There will be times when sticking to your routine seems easy, and other times when it seems like a hard chore. The longer you can stick with your regular routine the easier it will be to get back on track, if and when you falter.

6) Make a reasonable and realistic list of the reasons why you decided to start exercising and go back to it frequently. It might include such things as being able to climb stairs more easily, put shoes on more easily, or losing ten pounds. Periodically remind yourself how staying with an exercise regimen can help improve the quality of your life.

7) Keep progress reports or workout logs of your exercise sessions. There is nothing more motivating then seeing results. Benefits can appear as early as four to eight weeks. Within this time period you may notice that some everyday activities have become easier. If you look back at your workout log you may be surprised at how many more repetitions of each exercise you can now complete, or how much more aerobic activity you can tolerate. You may even have come close to accomplishing some of those goals in your list from item #6.

Special considerations for those with Multiple Sclerosis

➤ Do not overdo it. Throw out the "no pain, no gain" attitude. You can end up straining an already compromised muscular system, increasing pain and causing your body and mind to become overstressed, overworked, and overtired.
➤ Healthcare professionals, such as a physical or occupational therapists can help create a personal exercise program that meets your needs. The type of exercise that works best for you depends on your symptoms, fitness level, and overall health.

➤ Workout in a safe environment; avoid slippery floors, poor lighting, throw rugs, and other potential tripping hazards.
➤ If you have difficulty balancing, exercise within easy reach of a grab bar, chair, counter or railing.
➤ Watch out for overheating

Many people with MS experience a temporary worsening of their symptoms when they get too hot, such as getting overheated from exercise. This can occur with even a very slight elevation in core body temperature (one-quarter to one-half of a degree) because an elevated temperature, further impairs the ability of a demyelinated nerve to conduct electrical impulses. It is important to remember that heat generally produces only a temporary worsening of symptoms and does not cause more actual tissue damage. In most cases the symptoms usually rapidly resolve when the source of increased temperature is removed.

Tips for keeping cool
- Exercise in an air-conditioned room.
- Drink lots of cold fluids during exercise. Carry cold drinks in insulated containers that attach comfortably to a belt, waist-pack, backpack, or shoulder strap.
- Do not exercise during the hot time of the day. In warm weather avoid outdoor activities between 10:00 a.m. and 4:00 p.m.
- Become aware of your body. If you notice any symptoms that you didn't have before you began exercising, slow down or stop exercising until you cool down.
- Wear lightweight shoes. When the feet are cool, the rest of the body tends to be cool too.
- Wear vests, hats, or kerchiefs that hold "blue ice" gel packs or materials that can be chilled for long-lasting coolness.
- Dress in layers, in order to add or remove clothing as body temperature changes.
- Lower your body temperature immediately before and/or after exercise with a cool soak in a bathtub or shower. When no showers, tubs, pools, or gel packs are handy, try running cold water over your wrists for three to five minutes or apply cold paper towels to the neck and forehead.
- Refresh with "spritzes" of water from a plastic spray bottle – such as the type used for misting houseplants.

➤ Watch out for fatigue
A common symptom for those with MS is fatigue. You may find that you have more "off" days than "on" days. Also some medications can cause fatigue as a side effect.
Fatigue can also be related to respiratory problems. MS can sometimes affect breathing, and when it does, even simple activities can be tiring. This is especially true for people who have the most serious physical symptoms of MS. Lastly, sleep problems, problems falling asleep, staying asleep, or getting the right kind of sleep prevent people from feeling refreshed when they wake up.
Tips for handling fatigue

- Plan ahead. Get adequate sleep the night before engaging in exercise. Take a 15-minute nap a few hours preceding any demanding exercise.
- Schedule physical activity for the time of the day when energy is highest. Alternate more demanding exercise with activity requiring less.
- Always talk with exercise instructors about MS before starting a new class. This will allow the instructor to support you if you need to stop and rest.
- Apply the "2 minute rule": When feeling too sluggish for working out, commit to moderate exercise for just 2 minutes. The activity may generate the energy to continue. If fatigue persists, stop and rest.
- Avoid exhaustion. When it looks as if energy might start to fade, a 15-minute time-out may be all that's required to recharge. Lie or sit with eyes closed and breathe slowly and deeply. Do nothing, except possibly listen to soothing music or repeat a comforting word, sound, or phrase such as "I am calm."

Returning after an exacerbation

Attacks or exacerbations of MS may put exercise on the back burner. It may take as long as 6 weeks for strength and stamina to return to former levels after as little as one week of inactivity. Don't be discouraged. This is normal, even for people who do not have MS. Muscle mass can decrease noticeably after just one or two weeks of inactivity. When an exacerbation has interrupted an exercise routine, resume only after a doctor's OK. and prepare to be patient. It is not unusual for an exacerbation to cause a significant decrease in fitness level and physical capacity. It may take weeks or months to determine if a loss of function is permanent or not. If regular exercise has built up a reserve of strength, it will be easier to rebuild, even if some losses prove to be permanent. If the loss is not permanent, it is even possible to exceed one's former fitness level in time. When beginning to exercise again, set reasonable expectations. It is rarely possible to pick up a fitness program at the point where it was when the exacerbation began. Decreasing the intensity and/or the duration of an activity is a good way to get back into a routine.

Sometimes symptoms do not call for skipping an activity altogether, but do require making temporary alterations. Explaining this to class instructors ahead of time helps avoid embarrassment and allows the instructor to support your needs. Discuss any limitations that your MS is posing and ask about ways the activity might be modified. Do not be afraid to request that corrections or modifications be given in private before or after class. When exercising in a group setting, tell friends or teammates that MS is imposing some restrictions. Be specific. Explain, for example, that optic neuritis is making it difficult to see a ball, or that balance problems mean you will need to hold onto a chair or rail during the exercise session.

Remember, the most important thing is to exercise on a regular basis! Explore the suggestions and techniques written here and then work to find the best solution for your situation. Multiple Sclerosis affects each person differently. You are the best judge of what feels right for your body. Look at other sources of exercise and movement techniques. Try various approaches. Through experimentation you will find the routine that suits your needs and helps you to accomplish your goals.

Chapter One

Posture and Body Mechanics

You have to accept whatever comes and the only important thing is
that you meet it with the best you have to give.
- Eleanor Roosevelt

While adhering to a regular exercise routine can help manage the symptoms of many conditions, it is equally important to be mindful of how you use your body during everyday activities. If the goal is to improve posture, you should perform exercises that will strengthen and stretch those muscles that will help you reach that goal. However, if you then spend the rest of your day sitting incorrectly or lifting objects incorrectly, you may undo all of the benefits of your exercise session. Also, remember that incorrect posture and body mechanics can increase the chances of a fall. This chapter covers some of the basics concerning good posture and body mechanics.

Some typical activities during which we may use incorrect posture include:
➢ Sitting and watching TV
➢ Working at a computer
➢ Driving/riding in a car
➢ Looking downward while reading
➢ Household chores
➢ Yardwork

The following are some basic body mechanics principles to help correct posture, make everyday activities easier, and reduce the risk of falls.
➢ When bending, squat. Knees should be bent, back should be straight.
➢ Bend or hinge at the hips, not the waist.
➢ You are more steady with the feet wider apart and staggered. You are less steady with the feet closer together and parallel to each other.
➢ If lifting or bending compromises your balance, place your feet about hip width apart with one foot in front of the other for more stability.
➢ It is easier and more safe to push. It is harder and less safe to pull.
➢ Carry objects close to your body.
➢ When pushing or moving objects, use your body weight and momentum to push. Do not rely solely on arm strength.
➢ Lift with your legs, not your back.
➢ Always test the weight of the object before you try to lift it.
➢ Reorganize your house so that items you commonly use are within easy reach, preferably at a level between your knees and shoulders.
➢ Do not twist when lifting or pushing.
➢ When sweeping, vacuuming, shoveling, raking, etc., always face your work and move with it. Your nose, knees and toes should all be facing in the same direction.

➤ When performing the above mentioned activities, use a rocking motion, by transferring your weight from one leg to the other as you move. This allows your leg muscles to help with the work.

Many accidents happen in the kitchen and bathroom. Falls can happen while walking around, rising from a sitting position, and stepping out of the shower. The following are some tips for preventing falls.

➤ Be aware of the medications you take and their side effects. Some can increase the risk of falls.
➤ Try to avoid reaching out to furniture or handrails while walking. Stooping forward and reaching ahead of you can bring you out of balance and cause a fall.
➤ Be aware of uneven surfaces in rooms.
➤ Immediately wipe up any spilled liquids.
➤ Do not use scatter rugs that might slide on the floor. Secure them with skid-proof backing or securely tack them down. Worn or frayed rugs can cause tripping.
➤ If you need to use a step stool, make sure it is sturdy and secure.
➤ Always wear non-skid socks or slippers instead of regular socks.
➤ When rising from a lying down or a seated position, move slowly to avoid becoming dizzy.
➤ Make sure you have adequate lighting throughout the house. Use nightlights at night.
➤ Keep all floors clear of clutter.
➤ Before starting any activity, *think it through!* Make sure you place everything you need in an easy-to-get-to spot.
➤ Make a plan for getting help should you fall or become hurt.
➤ Try to locate phones throughout the house especially in areas such as the bathroom and kitchen where most accidents happen. As much as possible use cordless or cell phones you can carry with you. Make sure to place the phones at a level you can reach should you be unable to get up off the floor.
➤ Check in with someone on a regular basis in the event that you need help and are unable to get to a phone.
➤ Wear a medical alert bracelet or necklace if you fall frequently. With the push of a button, medical help will arrive quickly.

Hip Hinge

Before examining specific activities we will learn about a movement called the hip hinge. This involves reaching the buttocks back as if you were going to sit in a chair, bending at the knees, keeping a natural arch in the low back and coming forward by bending at the hips instead of the waist. This movement should be used when:

➢ Getting up and down from a chair
➢ Getting in and out of a car
➢ Lifting items off the floor and/or out of lower cabinets
➢ Shoveling, vacuuming, and cleaning
➢ Taking items in and out of an oven, washer, or dryer
➢ Anytime you need to stoop but cannot get down on one knee

Hip Hinge

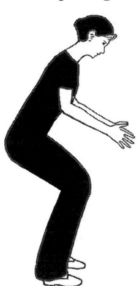

Correct Sitting Tips

➢ Avoid recliners. They promote rounding of the neck, shoulders and head, and also tightness in the hips.
➢ Avoid low, soft couches and chairs that make rising difficult.
➢ Choose a chair of average height with firm, smooth cushions and sturdy armrests. The height of the chair should allow for your hips and knees to be level with one another, or for the hips to be slightly higher than the knees.
➢ Keep your chin parallel to the floor.
➢ Avoid crossing your legs.
➢ Your computer screen and TV should be at eye level to minimize neck and eye strain.
➢ While reading, use a book stand or rest your elbows on a pillow or table.
➢ A good general rule is to change your posture every 15-20 minutes. At this point, get up and move around.
➢ Chairs should have a stable base. Swivel or rocking chairs are not a good choice because they can trigger a loss of balance and falling.
➢ To make it easier to stand up from a lower chair, raise the seat height by adding an extra cushion.
➢ Electric lift chairs and lift cushions can be helpful for people who have trouble getting out of chairs.

Correct Sitting Posture

➢ Ears over shoulders, shoulders over hips.
➢ Straight back allowing for the natural curve in the low back.
➢ Feet flat on the floor.
➢ Push the crown of the head to the ceiling, but keep your chin parallel to the floor.
➢ Abdominal muscles are lightly tucked in.
➢ Shoulders are down and relaxed.

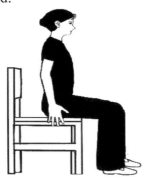

As much as you can throughout the day try to sit towards the front of the chair. This helps to prevent slouching. It also helps to strengthen the abdominal muscles by making them work to hold you up. Do not sit this way for too long at first. Try sitting this way for brief periods throughout the day, (when working at the computer and at the dinner table). Slowly increase the time you sit this way each day. When you need to sit back, slide the buttocks all the way back in the chair in order to keep the ears over the shoulders and the shoulders over hips. Avoid just leaning back and slouching in the chair.

Getting In and Out of a Chair

Falls often happen when moving from sitting to standing or standing to sitting. Protect your body and back by carefully lowering yourself in and lifting yourself out of chairs.

Sitting to Standing

✔ Bring your hips forward to the very edge of the chair (or couch) because it is more difficult to get up if you are sitting at the back of the chair.

✔ Feet should be approximately shoulder-width apart or wider to provide a good base of support.

✔ Position feet either parallel to each other or place your stronger leg slightly back.

Feet parallel.
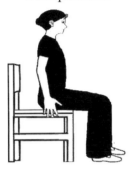

One leg slightly back.
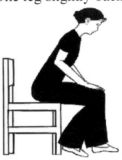

4. Lean forward at the hips until your head is positioned nose over knees and toes.

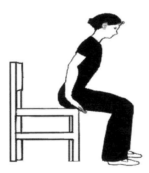

5. Continue to lean forward, bringing the nose over the toes to come up to standing. Let your legs do most of the work. Try to push off of your thighs to get up. Your leg muscles are much larger and stronger than those in your arms. If your legs are not strong enough to lift you up, you can push off the seat or arms of the chair, but avoid relying on arm strength alone to lift yourself up.

6. Keep your back straight, head up, eyes forward.

Getting up pushing off of your thighs

Getting up pushing off of the seat of the chair

Getting up pushing off of the arms of a chair

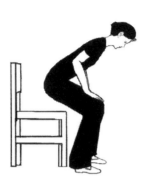 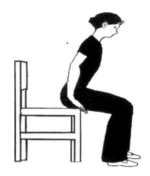 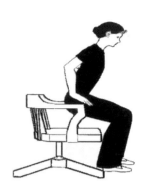

Standing to Sitting

1. Take large rather then short shuffling steps as you approach the chair.
2. Position yourself so the chair is centered directly behind you. You should feel the chair against the back of your legs before sitting.
3. Reach back for the seat or armrests as you "hip hinge" forward. Again think nose over knees and toes.
5. Keep your back straight, head up and eyes forward.
    Do not reach for the chair before you turn to sit; you might lose your balance or fall.
6. Use your leg strength to lower your body *slowly and gently* to the edge of the chair. Then slide back. If your legs are not strong enough to lower yourself to the chair, use your arms to help control your descent. *Never* crash down into a chair. Crashing down into a chair can cause injury to the back and oftentimes triggers a fall.

Sitting down using the seat of the chair   Sitting down using the arms of a chair

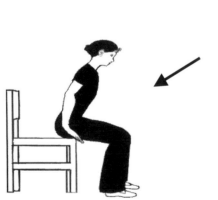 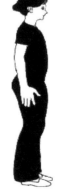 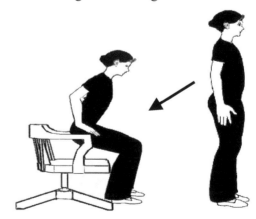

Getting In and Out of a Car

To get into a car

➤ Avoid stepping from a curb into a car, or from a car onto a curb. Remember always; from ground level to car, from car to ground level.
➤ Avoid getting into a car sideways (placing one leg or foot in first).

1. Approach the car seat the same way you would a chair. Turn and back in towards the seat with your buttocks leading the way.
2. Reach back for the seat or dashboard and slowly lower yourself to sit at the edge. Never hold on to the door which can move and trigger a fall.
3. With one hand hold onto the seat inside the car. With the other hand lift one leg at a time into the car. Then you can turn your body on the seat to face forward.

➤ Place a plastic bag on cloth seats to make turning easier.

To get out of a car

➤ Avoid getting out of a car sideways.

1. Hold onto the dashboard with one hand. With the other hand, lift one leg at a time out of the car.
2. Then you can turn your body on the seat to face out.
3. Your body should be in the car and both of your legs should be out of the car and both feet flat on the ground.
4. Then, move the buttocks forward to the edge of the car seat and lean forward (hip hinge) while pushing up from the seat or dashboard.

➤ Never pull up on the car door, which can move and trigger a fall.

Correct Standing Tips

➢ Keep your chin parallel to the floor.
➢ Maintain a broad base of support by keeping your feet shoulder width apart or wider.
➢ Abdominal muscles should be in, shoulders back and down, head and chest up, and knees slightly bent, but never locked.
➢ An easy way to help you stand straight is to think about lifting the top of your head to the ceiling. Do not lift your chin, your chin stays parallel with the floor. As you focus on lifting the top of the head up, you may feel yourself standing taller as your abdominal and waist muscles tighten.

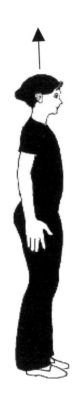

Correct Walking

> Do not look straight down while walking. Instead look ahead and slightly down. Look down with your eyes, not your head.
> As much as possible, keep your hands free. Carry light loads in small body packs.
> If balance or strength is affecting your ability to walk, use a mobility aid (cane, walker or walking stick), adjusted to the proper height.
> When stepping make sure you flex your front foot, letting your heel strike first. Walking with a shuffle or stepping on the toes first is often the cause of falls. Flexing the foot and landing with the heel first and toes up forces you to pick up your feet, lessening the risk of tripping and falling.
> When you walk make sure you swing your arms. When stepping, swing the arm that is opposite to the forward foot. Swing the arm up to shoulder height. This walking technique will aid in maintaining balance, reduce the risk of falls, and it provides momentum.

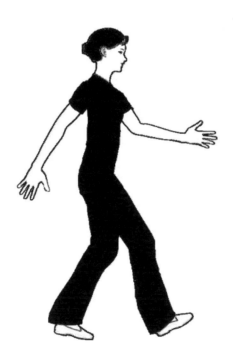

Lying Down and Getting In and Out of Bed

It is not unusual to have trouble turning over, or getting in and out of bed. Lying on your back with a soft pillow under the knees, or on your side with a soft pillow between the knees are the best postures for sleeping. It is also good to avoid using too many pillows, or too thin of a pillow under the head. Avoid sleeping in a chair. When napping lie down so that the head and neck are supported.

Tips for rolling or turning over in bed
- A satin sheet or piece of satin material tucked across the middle of the bed makes it easier to turn over.
- Flannel sheets and heavy blankets can make it more difficult to turn over.
- When turning, bend your knees and put your feet flat on the bed. Allow the knees to fall to one side as you begin to roll. Turn your head in the direction you are rolling and reach the top arm across the body.
- A straight back chair anchored at the side of the bed or a bed rail can help you roll more easily.

Tips for scooting over in bed
- Bend your knees placing the feet flat on the bed.
- Push into the bed with the feet and hands to lift the hips up. Then shift the hips in the desired direction.
- Finish by repositioning the feet in the direction your hips moved.

Helpful bedroom aids
- A helping handle or bed rail that attaches between the mattress and box spring provides assistance with rolling, and support for pushing yourself to an upright position. An inexpensive alternative to a bed rail is a straight-back chair securely laced to the bed frame.
- An adjustable blanket support keeps the blanket off feet, making it easier to move.
- A motion-activated nightlight detects movement and automatically switches on.
- Electric beds make it easy to elevate your head and upper body, making breathing easier.

Getting Into Bed

1. Approach the bed as you would a chair; feel the mattress behind both legs. Reach back for the bed with your hands.
2. Slowly lower yourself to a seated position on the edge of the bed using your leg muscles to control your descent. Use the hip hinge motion (pg. 19).

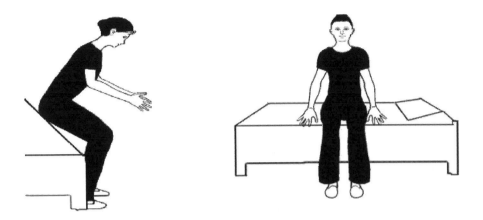

3. As your trunk goes down, bring the legs up (like a seesaw motion).

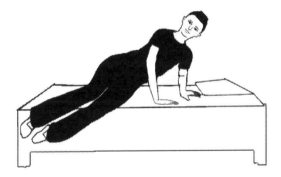

4. Use your arms to lower yourself onto your side and then roll to your back.

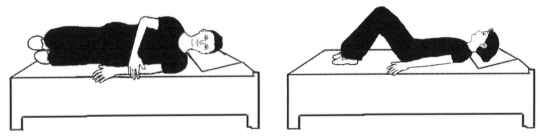

Getting Out of Bed

Reverse the order of the above steps to get out of bed.

1. Bend the knees and place your feet flat on the bed. Reach across with the top arm and turn your head to look in the direction you are rolling. Let the knees fall to the side so the body moves as a unit. Roll all the way onto your side toward the edge of the bed

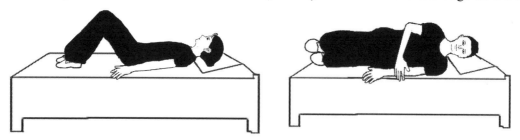

2. Push with your arms to lift the body up. As your body comes up, let the legs slide off the side of the bed.

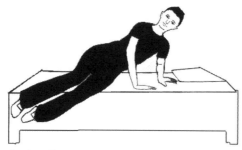

4. Lower the feet towards the floor as you push with your arms into a sitting position. Slide to the edge of the bed and use your legs to come to standing. Use the hip hinge motion (pg. 19).

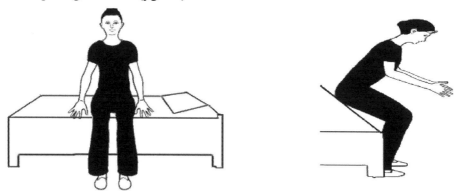

Avoid coming to a sitting position directly from your back. This strains the back muscles and is a more difficult way to get up. It is much safer to roll to your side before coming to a seated position.

Bathing, Grooming and Toileting

Bathing

Since shower stalls are easier to get into and out of than bathtubs, they are usually better for bathing. If you must use a bathtub, a tub transfer bench will help you get in and out more easily. Shower chairs allow you to sit in the shower while you bathe. Putting on a terry robe after bathing also makes drying easier.

➢ Bathtubs and shower stalls should have at least two grab bars to hold on to as you get in and out.
➢ Grab bars should always be professionally installed.
➢ *Never* use the towel bar, soap dish, or faucet as a handrail. They are not secure enough to hold your body weight.
➢ If you sit on a tub transfer bench or shower chair while showering, use a hand-held showerhead. This will allow you to sit first and then hold the showerhead to direct the water away from you so you can adjust the temperature safely.
➢ All bathtubs and shower stalls should have a non-skid rubber bath mat. All bath rugs should have a rubber backing.
➢ Be careful when using bar soap. It is slippery, hard to hold, and when dropped leaves a slippery film on the floor. Try pump soaps or soap-on-a-rope.
➢ Keep a nightlight on in the bathroom.
➢ If alone, bring a cordless or cell phone into the bathroom with you so that you can call for help if you need it. Make sure you put the phone in a place you can easily reach from the floor, should you fall.

Grooming

The stiffness and tremor common with MS can make it difficult to handle toothbrushes, razors and hairdryers. These tips may help.

➢ Sit down to brush your teeth, shave, or dry your hair. Sitting not only reduces the risk of falling, but also helps conserve your energy. A shower or commode chair works well for this. Leave the doors underneath the sink open to make room for your knees.
➢ Use a hands-free hairdryer that can be mounted on a vanity.

Helpful bathing and toileting aids

➢ A tub transfer bench or shower chair with a back adds extra safety for those who tire easily.
➢ An extra-long hand-held shower spray allows you to shower while seated on a bath chair or in the tub.
➢ Commode frames make it easier to sit down on and get up from the toilet. Raised toilet seats also work.
➢ Lever faucet adapters ease grasping and turning.

➢ A long-handled sponge or brush helps people with limited range of motion reach the back and legs.

Remember to think about your body mechanics during all activities. For example, when brushing your teeth, try to avoid rounding the back when using the sink. Keep the back straight and bend the knees instead.

<table>
<tr><td align="center">Correct
Knees bent, back straight.</td><td align="center">Incorrect
Knees locked, back and
shoulders rounded.</td></tr>
</table>

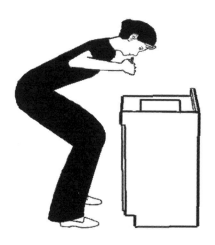 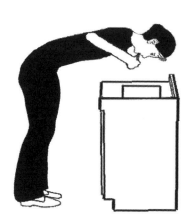

Dressing

General tips for dressing

➢ Allow plenty of time for dressing. Hurrying can lead to stress and frustration which can slow you down.
➢ Sit down when dressing. Choose a chair with firm support and arms. Do not sit on the edge of the bed to dress because this can lead to loss of balance and falling.
➢ Choose clothing with fewer buttons, zippers, and other closures that might be difficult to use.
➢ Replace buttons by sewing on touch fasteners such as Velcro®.
➢ Try loose fitting clothing made of stretchy fabric which is easy to put on.
➢ Bedroom slippers which can slide off your feet should be replaced with non-skid socks.
➢ Lightweight, supportive shoes with Velcro® closures, elastic shoelaces, or "curly fries" shoelaces make it easier to put on and take off shoes.
➢ An extra-long shoehorn helps shoes slide on without your having to bend over.

Remember to think about your body mechanics while dressing. For example; when putting on your shoes avoid rounding forward, and instead either bring a foot up to your knee or put your foot on a footstool.

Correct	**Correct**	**Incorrect**
Back straight, shoulders down.	Bringing your leg up instead of bending forward.	Back and shoulders rounded forward.

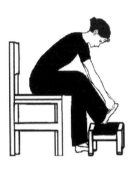 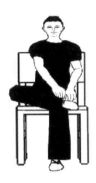 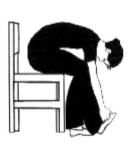

Household tasks

During housework and yard work it is easy to slip into poor postural habits. Below are some guidelines to help you maintain posture and avoid falls.

➢ It is safer and easier to push rather than pull.
➢ If standing for long periods at a sink, counter, or workbench, try putting one foot up on a stool.
➢ When vacuuming, sweeping, or raking, always face your work. Nose, knees, and toes should all be facing in the same direction. Try to avoid twisting and bending in order to protect your back.
➢ Use a rocking motion transferring weight from one foot to the other, thereby relying on your body weight to do the work instead of your back.

Correct	**Incorrect**	**Incorrect**
Back straight; knees bent. Broom is close to body, facing work.	Back and shoulders rounded, knees locked. Broom too far away.	Twisting back and knees. Nose, knees, and toes not facing broom

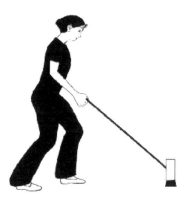 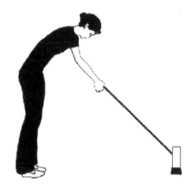 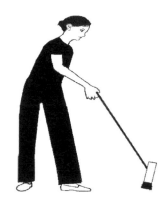

Correct	**Incorrect**
Correct way to sit at computer. Back straight, shoulders down. Screen at eye level.	Incorrect way to sit. Screen too high, wrists are bent

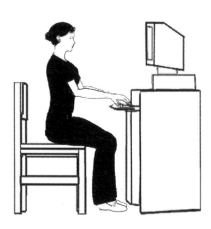 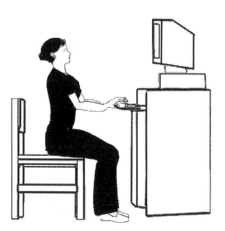

✓   When lifting always bend your knees and lift with your legs, not your back. Always test the weight of the object you are going to lift. Keep the object close to your body, and again face your work. Remember to use the hip hinge (pg. 19). Instead of rounding through the back, bend the knees, and reach the buttocks back (as if you were about to sit in a chair). Feet can be about hip width apart or wider if needed for balance. Use this motion regardless of how heavy or light the object is. Many back injuries occur just by moving the wrong way or when lifting light objects!

Correct	**Incorrect**	**Correct**
Back straight, bending at hips. Stand close to the object and use your legs to lift.	Back rounded, bending at waist. Object too far away, using back to lift.	Correct way to carry. Keep item close to your body.

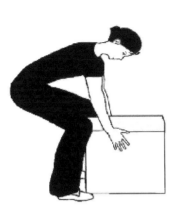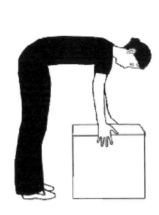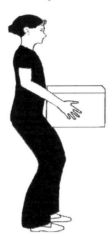

Correct way to reach items in low places. Get down and close to the object.

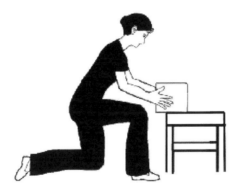

Another method which can be used to pick items up off the floor is called the golfer's reach. This movement is sometimes used by golfers to pick up the ball. Make sure you hold onto something sturdy to avoid losing your balance. Tip the upper body forward as you lift the back leg. This keeps your back straight versus bending at the waist or rounding the upper back.

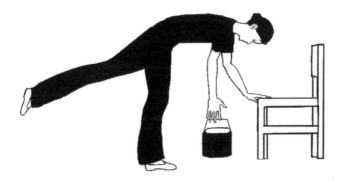

It is also important to think about how you reach items that are higher up. If an item is above shoulder height it is best to use a sturdy step stool.

Incorrect

Overreaching from shoulder, not a sturdy stance. Increased risk for falling backwards or dropping the item.

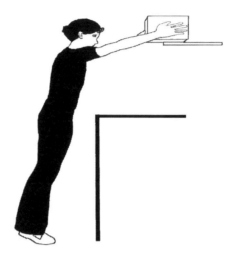

Correct

Place the item on a counter before stepping up onto or off of the stool. *Never* climb up or step down from a stool with items in your hands! Keep the item close to you and get as close as you can to the shelf

.

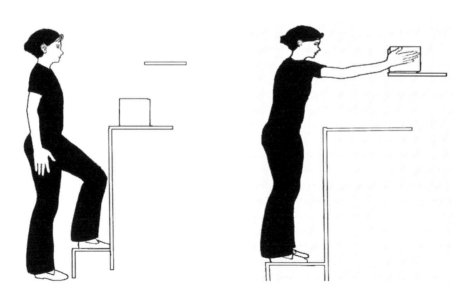

Getting Down on the Floor

If you practice getting up and down from the floor on a regular basis, you will be more likely to be able to get up without help should you fall. People who fall at home must sometimes wait hours or even days before help arrives. When first attempting this, make sure you have someone around to help you until you can easily get up alone.

1. First make sure there is a sturdy chair nearby. Use the hip hinge motion (pg. 19) to place your hands on the chair.

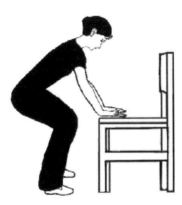

2. Then place one knee (whichever knee is more comfortable to do this with) on the floor. Continue to use the chair for support. Then come down on to all fours and move the chair away a bit.

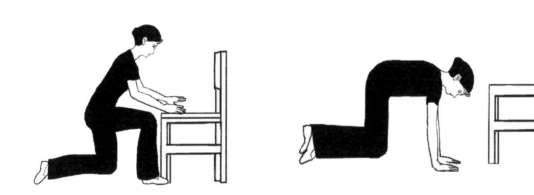

3. Then lower yourself down onto one hip, (whichever hip is more comfortable to bear weight on).

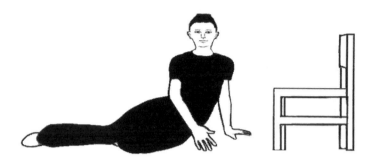

4. Next, lower yourself down so that you are lying on your side.

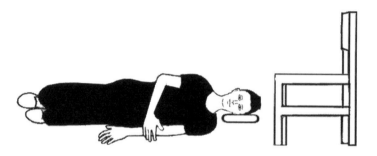

5. From here you can roll over onto your back.

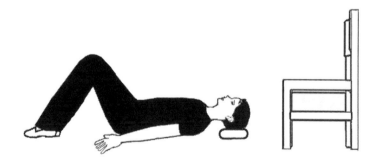

Getting Up From the Floor

1. Make sure there is a chair or sturdy piece of furniture near by.
   If you have fallen in the middle of a room, crawl or scoot yourself over to
   something sturdy.

2. If you are on your back, first roll onto one side, (whichever side is more
   comfortable to bear weight on). Roll your body as a unit, the same as when
   getting out of bed (pg. 28).

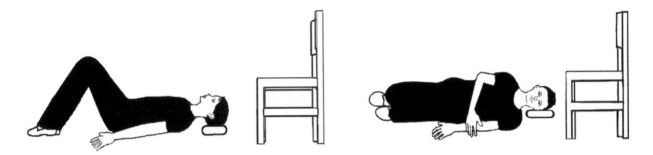

3. Then, using your arms, push up onto your hip.

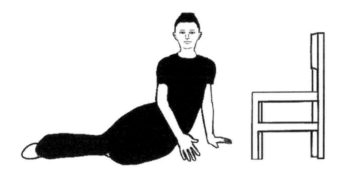

4. Next come up to all fours.

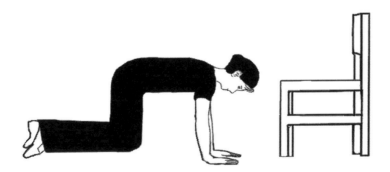

5. Bring one foot forward so that you are on one knee (whichever knee is more comfortable to do this with). Place your hands on the chair for support.

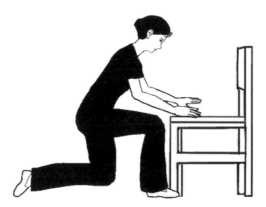

6. Using the chair for support, use the hip hinge motion to come up to standing. Remember to keep your back straight when transitioning from kneeling to standing.

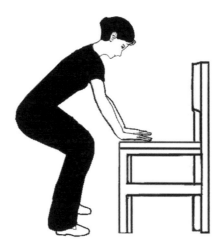

Summary

Begin to incorporate correct body mechanics techniques on a daily basis. At first it may seem like daily tasks take longer, but with more practice using correct body mechanics will become more natural. With time, you may find that you automatically correct yourself, and eventually it will become common practice to use good working habits.

To fully manage your symptoms and remain active, using correct body mechanics is an important step. Taking the time to do things correctly and safely will help to reduce the risk of falls and keep your back and joints safe from injury. Many falls and accidents happen as the result of rushing and not thinking our actions through. Taking the time to do things correctly helps avoid accidents enabling you to stay independent longer.

If you are experiencing significant difficulty with any of your daily activities, talk with your healthcare provider about attending physical or occupational therapy. Physical and occupational therapists are specially trained to work with you and your individual situation to help make everyday activities safer and more enjoyable.

Chapter Two

Diaphragmatic Breathing and Aerobic Exercise

*"Our greatest glory is not in never falling, but
in rising every time we fall."*
- Confucius

One component of an exercise regimen is aerobic or cardiovascular exercise. This type of exercise includes any activity that is sustained and raises the heart and breathing rate. The purpose of aerobic exercise is to strengthen the heart and lungs, train the body to utilize oxygen more efficiently, and help maintain a healthy weight and blood pressure.

Examples of aerobic activities include:
➢ Walking
➢ Biking
➢ Aerobic dancing

Regular aerobic exercise can help:
➢ Take off excess weight and maintain a healthy weight
➢ Strengthen the heart and lungs
➢ Improve stamina and endurance
➢ Reduce stress
➢ Improve mood and combat depression
➢ Help control high blood pressure and high cholesterol

Current guidelines suggest that all adults should get at least 30 minutes of moderate intensity aerobic exercise at least 5 days a week. If you have not been exercising regularly, this would be too much to start with. If you are just beginning to exercise either for the first time, or after being away from it for a while, try for 5-10 minutes two to three times per week. Then, each week try to add one to two minutes until you can comfortably do 15 minutes three times per week. From there keep adding more and more time slowly, and eventually add additional days. A common mistake made by many is to start off too vigorously. This leads to muscle soreness and fatigue, making it difficult to keep exercising. Starting slowly and increasing gradually, allows the body to adapt to the exercise. While you may feel some stiffness or soreness initially, your routine should not cause pain or discomfort to the point where it restricts you from doing daily activities.

Before beginning aerobic exercise, make sure you warm-up by taking a short walk, or performing the "rhythmic limbering" exercises included in this chapter. The goal of aerobic exercise is to raise the heart and breathing rate to a point where you will benefit from the routine. During aerobic classes it is commonly recommended to take your pulse (or your heart rate) during the exercise session, with a goal of sustaining it at a level equal to 60 to 80 percent of your heart's maximum ability. However, many medications can interfere with your heart rate. For example some heart medications work to keep your heart rate lower. When you start exercising the medication will continue to try to lower your heart rate. This means you may be working out very hard, but your medication is constantly lowering your heart rate. If you continue to try to increase your heart rate to 60 to 80 percent, you may be putting yourself at risk for injury. In other words, taking your heart rate may not be providing you with an accurate picture of how hard you are actually working. Another concern with taking your heart rate is that many people have a hard time locating their pulse. This may require you to stop exercising while trying to find your pulse. Stopping causes your heart rate to drop, which interferes with keeping the exercise at a steady pace.

Given this, many people choose to use a scale known as the Rating of Perceived Exertion. This scale assigns a number to describe how hard you feel you are working. It is a self-rating technique you can do periodically during your routine to judge if you are working at the right level to gain benefits. At periods throughout your routine take a moment to use the following scale to rate how you are doing.

The Rating of Perceived Exertion scale is as follows:

1   No effort, resting
2   Very, Very Light
3   Very Light
4   Fairly Light
5   Moderate
6   Somewhat Hard
7   Hard
8   Very Hard
9   Very, Very Hard
10 Maximum Effort

For your aerobic program, you should gradually work up to a level between 5-7. Working at a level of 1-4 will not be vigorous enough to get the full benefit from your routine. Working above level 7 may lead to soreness, injury and fatigue. Another way to test how hard you are working is the talk test. While exercising you should not be so out of breath that you can not even answer a yes or no question. If you are gasping for breath just to say a few words you are working too hard. If on the other hand you are able to carry on a full conversation with no trouble, you may not be exercising hard enough.

Using music for the aerobic component helps to ensure that you are working at a good pace in order to raise your heart rate high enough to get benefits. It also can make the time go by faster. Using music is also a good way to time your routine. However long you are aiming to exercise - five minutes, ten minutes, or a longer amount of time - try making a tape or CD that plays the same amount of time you want your routine to be. In the classes we teach, our music is approximately 120 beats per minute.
To determine the beats per minute of a song do the following:

- ➢ Get a stopwatch or watch with a second hand
- ➢ Play the music you wish to use
- ➢ Tap to the beat of the song with your hand or foot
- ➢ Count how many times you tap in a 15-second period
- ➢ You should count about 30 beats. (30 x 4 is 120). We times this number by 4, as there are four 15-second periods per minute

If you find that this speed of music too fast to keep up with, start with slower music and gradually work up to music that is 120 beats per minute.

The following movements are the ones we teach in our program. They move the body in a variety of directions to fully work the joints and muscles. Challenging the body to travel in different directions such as forward, backwards, and sideways helps to improve balance. Because there are many other ways to move the body, you may wish to vary this routine with other movements you know. The aerobic exercises can be done standing, standing and holding onto a chair or counter for support, or while seated on a physioball or chair. *Try to do as much as you can standing.* This will help you to improve your balance and standing provides weight bearing exercise to help strengthen the bones, as well as improving your cardiovascular health.

Experiment with the different variations to find the right option for you. You can do some of each. For example, if you are new to exercise or having a day when you are not feeling well, you may choose to do a few minutes standing, and then a few minutes seated. As with everything in this program explore different approaches to see what feels best. The movements will be shown one per page with instructions. The last page will list all the movements together and provides sample sequences so you can move through your routine more smoothly.

It is important to let the body cool down slowly after exercise. After completing aerobic activity, continue with some type of gentle movement for another three to five minutes to let the heart and breathing rate slowly adjust back to their pre-exercise level.

Tips for those with MS

When it comes to exercise, having MS presents challenges. It's important to work within individual abilities and to stay attuned to new needs as symptoms or medications change. Some people with MS will experience numbness, tingling, or blurred vision when they exercise and some find that exercise actually worsens symptoms of spasticity. This can be relieved or reduced with a gentle warm-up. These symptoms are usually temporary and decline shortly after stopping. However it is safer to go easy at first until you know how exercise affects you.

It is also common to over do it. This can lead to fatigue and increased possibility of injury. Start slowly and add additional time gradually with each session. People with MS can increase their endurance just as anyone else can, if it is approached sensibly. Studies show that exercisers with MS who work more slowly at the beginning achieve more in the end.

Remember:

➢ Take approximately five minutes to warm up before aerobic exercise.
➢ Drink juice or water before beginning and after finishing.
➢ Deep breathing is important for building lung capacity. Use deep diaphragmatic breathing during both warm-up and exercise periods. (pg. 50).
➢ Take approximately five minutes to cool down at the end
  Cool down by repeating the activity at a gradually decreasing pace for two to three minutes. Stop and gently stretch the muscles you have used.
➢ Rest following exercise. Fatigue that lingers after 1 hour of rest is a sign of having overextended.
➢ Avoid overheating.

Other aerobic exercise options

➢ Exercise in the water. Exercising in cool water is ideal for those with MS. Water prevents overheating, and its natural buoyancy gives support, making movement easier. Water exercise allows you to move in ways you might not be able to on land. All of the exercises shown in this book can also be done in the water.

➢ Adjustable-speed treadmills offer the benefits of walking in a comfortable environment. Using a treadmill with handrails in an air-conditioned room overcomes the challenges of outdoor heat and humidity, uneven paths, and uphill climbs.

➢ Other types of equipment include stair steppers, stationary bicycles, and cross-country ski machines. Upright or recumbent bikes can work both the arms and legs. Visit a store and actually try the equipment before buying it to make sure it is comfortable to use and so that you know how to adjust it to fit your specific needs and limits.

➢ Exercise with a physioball. All of the warm-up and aerobic exercises in this book are shown while sitting on a physioball. Some with MS experience pain in the bottom of their feet which makes standing aerobics too uncomfortable. However, chair exercises are often not vigorous enough. Working out on a ball takes pressure off of your feet and it provides a good cardiovascular workout.

Physioballs are heavy-duty, inflatable balls that come in many sizes and shapes and can be used to create a full body workout. They are designed to hold up to 400 to 700 pounds. Physioballs are comfortable, supportive and they conform to your unique anatomy. They also make it easier to perform different exercises in many different positions. Working with a physioball is a great way to tone and strengthen your entire body including the abs and lower back. They are especially beneficial for those living with back and/or joint pain since they take pressure off of the feet and joints, making exercise more tolerable. Many of our students who can not do traditional aerobics or strength training exercises find that they can do a complete hour long workout on the ball. In general physioballs offer you a fun, safe, and highly effective way to exercise.

Working on the ball is also a very effective way to improve balance. Maintaining proper alignment on the ball stimulates the body's nervous and muscular system as well as the reflexes. It also encourages the body to react as a whole and integrated unit in order to maintain correct posture and balance. When using the ball correctly, the body is required to utilize many muscles for stabilization. Even while training other muscle groups, the abdominal and back muscles must work to balance and stabilize the body. This process strengthens the muscles that help you to maintain good posture which is important for relieving and preventing low back pain. Exercising on an unstable base such as a physioball, will help strengthen your core while providing you with many different angles to work from. Since exercising on a physioball can be challenging, it is best to hold onto a chair or counter at first, until you get your balance on the ball.

Physioballs come in different sizes and should be purchased according to your body height. Measure the ball from top to bottom (diameter).

Your Height	Ball Size
5' 3" and under	55 cm
5' 4" to 5' 10"	65 cm
5' 11" to 6' 4"	75 cm
6' 5" and over	85 cm

Exploring the Cardiovascular and Circulatory System.
Why I need to exercise my heart

The cardiovascular system is made up of the heart, blood, and blood vessels. The circulatory system is your body's delivery system. Blood leaving the heart delivers oxygen and nutrients to every part of the body. On the way back to the heart, the blood picks up and carries away waste products.

The heart

The heart is a very important muscle of the body. In an average lifetime the heart beats more than two and a half billion times and is often described as a pump. It pumps blood around your body supplying the cells with nutrients and removing waste. It contracts on average between 60 - 80 times a minute, more if you are exercising or exerting yourself. This number is known as your "heart rate." An adult's heart pumps nearly 4000 gallons of blood each day. The heart contains four chambers, and is shaped and sized roughly like a man's fist. The top two chambers are called the atria and the bottom two chambers are called the ventricles.

Aorta - Carries oxygenated blood to the body.

Superior Vena Cava

Right Atrium – Receives blood from the body

Right Ventricle – Pumps blood to the lungs to be oxygenated

Inferior Vena Cava

Pulmonary Artery – Carries blood to the lungs

Pulmonary Veins

Left Atrium – Receives oxygenated blood from the lungs

Left Ventricle – Pumps oxygenated blood to the body

Septum

Blood Pressure

Blood pressure measures the pressure the blood exerts against the walls of the arteries. This pressure changes constantly according to the body's needs. As the ventricles contract, the pressure measured is called the systolic pressure. As the ventricles relax, the pressure measured is called the diastolic blood pressure. The average systolic blood pressure is 100 to 140 mmHg (mm of mercury). The average diastolic pressure is 60 to 85 mmHg. This determines the blood pressure, which is recorded as a fraction such as 120/80 mmHg.

Exercise and your heart

Regular aerobic exercise is the best method of keeping the heart muscle strong and healthy as it places specific demands on the body. During aerobic exercise the muscles demand more oxygen-rich blood and give off more carbon dioxide and other waste. To accomplish this the heart must beat faster, and pump more blood with each beat to meet these demands. This means that your heart rate and blood pressure must increase in order to supply the working muscles with an increased need for blood and oxygen.

The effects of regular exercise will depend on the type, duration, frequency and intensity of training. Since the heart muscle must work harder to accommodate the increased needs during exercise, the heart muscle will become stronger and more efficient. When you give your heart this kind of workout on a regular basis your heart will become better at its main job, delivering blood and oxygen to all parts of your body. When you follow a program of regular aerobic exercise, over time your heart grows stronger and can meet the muscles' demands without as much effort.

Regular aerobic exercise can:
➤ Increase the size of major coronary vessels, making it easier for the blood to flow to all regions of the heart - in other words there is more space and less resistance for the blood to flow through as it travels throughout the body
➤ Increase the size and pumping ability of the heart - as with all of the muscles in the body, when the heart muscle is stressed through exercise it gets stronger
➤ Increase the number of capillaries in the body thereby aiding in the distribution of blood
➤ Lower blood pressure due to a stronger more efficient system
➤ Lead to a decrease in body fat and weight, so there is less area for the body to have to supply blood to
➤ Lower resting heart rate, meaning that the heart will not have to work as hard at rest

Regular aerobic exercise produces a more efficient system that recovers quicker. This means that when you stop the aerobic exercise session your blood pressure, rate of breathing, and heart rate will return to their pre-exercise levels more quickly then they could before you started an exercise program. This means that your body is adapting to the exercise program and is becoming more efficient.

Exploring the Respiratory System
Why I need to exercise my lungs

You breathe with the help of your diaphragm and other muscles in your chest and abdomen. These muscles literally change the space and pressure inside the body to accommodate breathing. Your lungs are like a pair of balloons that expand when you inhale. When you inhale, your diaphragm drops down so the lung cavity can expand and take in air. When you exhale the muscles squeeze your rib cage, your diaphragm moves upwards, your lungs begin to collapse, and the air is pushed up and out of your body.

How the oxygen you breathe gets into the blood

You breathe in about 20 times per minute. Every minute you inhale approximately 13 pints of air. In the course of a day, approximately 8,000 to 9,000 liters of inhaled air meets 8,000 to 10,000 liters of blood pumped in by the heart through the pulmonary artery (see pg. 45).

The air you inhale passes through the nasal passages that filter, heat, and moisten the air before it flows into the back of the throat. The air then flows down through the trachea (windpipe) to where the lower ribs meet the center of your chest. Here your windpipe divides into two tubes, which lead to the lungs. Inside each of your lungs tubes called bronchi branch into still even smaller tubes much like the branches of a tree. At the end of these tubes are millions of tiny sacs called alveoli. Here, the red blood cells interact with these sacs to trade in the old carbon dioxide that your body's cells have made, for some new oxygen you have just breathed in.

The "new" oxygen passes through the walls of each alveoli into the tiny capillaries that surround them and enters the blood, where it is carried by red blood cells to the heart. The heart then sends the oxygen-rich blood through arteries and capillaries to all the cells in the body.

Veins then carry the oxygen-depleted blood back to the heart and then into the lungs. Here, the carbon dioxide and waste picked up by the alveoli travels through the lungs, back up your windpipe and it is expelled with every exhale.

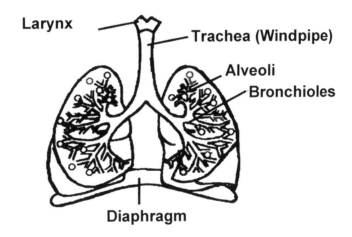

Larynx   **Trachea (Windpipe)**   **Alveoli**   **Bronchioles**   **Diaphragm**

Exercise and your respiratory system

During exercise the muscles use more oxygen than when they are at rest. At rest the muscles take up 6 ml per 100 ml of oxygen. During heavy exercise the muscles can take up as much as 17 ml per 100 ml. Aerobic exercise places demands on the system which results in a stronger respiratory system, making it more efficient at delivering and processing oxygen in the body.

Cardiorespiratory endurance (the health of our heart and lungs) refers to the body's ability to sustain prolonged activity. The endurance of this system can be tested by measuring the highest rate of oxygen consumption attainable during maximal exertion. This level of maximal exertion is known as your "VO2 max." When you reach this level your body can no longer deliver oxygen as quickly as your muscles need to receive it. Thus you will not be able to continue the activity you were doing for much longer. Regular aerobic activity has been shown to increase this level, allowing you to perform activities for longer periods at a higher intensity.

Regular aerobic exercise brings about changes in the body's cardiorespiratory system enabling it to function more effectively. Much like the heart during exercise, aerobic exercise forces the lungs to work harder and faster to deliver the needed oxygen, which strengthens and conditions them. Exercise is good for every part of your body, especially your lungs and heart. As you breathe more deeply and take in more air, your lungs become stronger and more efficient at supplying your body with the air it needs for exercise and everyday activities.

Below are some of the benefits of regular aerobic exercise.

➢ Makes your heart and cardiorespiratory system stronger and more efficient.
➢ Improves lung capacity. This is very beneficial for those with MS. An increase in lung capacity means that you do not get out of breath as quickly during all types of activity such as climbing stairs and walking uphill.
➢ Strengthens the diaphragm muscle.
➢ Decreases fatigue. After approximately four to eight weeks of participating in regular aerobic exercise you may notice that you feel less tired during exercise and everyday activities.
➢ Induces sleep. Many of our class participants who do regular aerobic exercise notice that they sleep better at night.
➢ Increases your tolerance for exercise. You will find you can exercise longer and at a harder pace then when you started.

Diaphragmatic Breathing

Before beginning to explore different movement techniques it is important to discuss breathing. Most people take shallow breaths moving only the chest and shoulders. When taking shallow breaths the diaphragm is not used to its full capacity. It is more efficient and beneficial to learn to breathe more deeply, using the diaphragm. MS can cause a decrease in lung capacity, leading to fatigue, so regular deep breathing is essential.

Learning to breathe abdominally (from the diaphragm) also helps to promote relaxation, which improves physical and mental health. This occurs since belly breathing is a more efficient way for the body to take in oxygen and remove carbon dioxide.

The diaphragm is a large, dome-shaped muscle that contracts rhythmically and continually, and most of the time involuntarily. The diaphragm sits beneath the lungs and above the abdominal cavity. When you exhale the abdominal muscles should contract, allowing the diaphragm to move upward, so the air is fully expelled from the lungs. During inhalation the abdominal muscles should relax and move outwards, allowing the diaphragm muscle to move downward, so the lungs can fully expand.

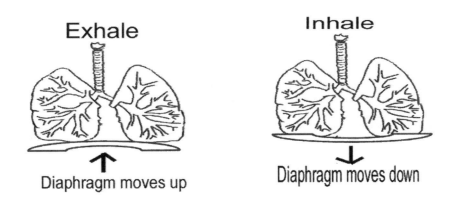

Although breathing is an automatic function, the movements of the diaphragm can be controlled voluntarily with training. Benefits of diaphragmatic breathing include:

➢ A more efficient exchange of oxygen and carbon dioxide
➢ Promotion of general relaxation
➢ Improved circulation
➢ Removal of waste products from the blood
➢ Slower heart rate and breathing rate
➢ Calming of the mind

This method of breathing may feel awkward because we were often taught to pull in the stomach muscles as we inhale, but this actually restricts the movement of the diaphragm. However, with practice this deeper form of breathing will become more natural. The easiest way to practice diaphragmatic breathing is lying down, the second easiest is while standing, and most difficult is while seated. You can begin to try this deep breathing by lying on your bed or couch. Then try it while standing, and then seated. We will use this breath during every exercise and movement in this book.

Diaphragmatic breathing should be done as much as possible through the nose rather than the mouth. Breathing through the nose is more efficient and relaxing for the body because the nasal cavity is better designed to purify and warm the air. If you are experiencing any type of respiratory or sinus concerns, or if you become dizzy while breathing strictly through the nose, try inhaling only through the nose and then exhaling through pursed lips.

Belly Breathing Lying Down

Lie on your back with a pillow under your head if needed. Place one hand on your belly and the other on your chest. As you exhale through the nose gently contract the abdominal muscles and push all of the air out of your belly and lungs. The hand on the belly should move down. Think of moving the belly towards the floor.

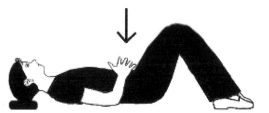

As you inhale through the nose let the abdominal muscles relax and let the belly rise first. With the inhalation the hand on the belly should move up and the hand on the chest should stay still. Think of moving the belly towards the ceiling. Then let the chest and the hand on the chest rise. It may take some practice to have the belly move first, or at all.

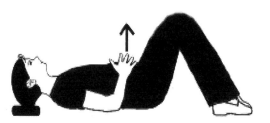

Belly Breathing Seated

Use correct sitting posture.
Sit at the front edge of the chair and away from the back of the chair.
Feet should be flat on the floor.
The shoulders stay down and relaxed.
Place one hand on your belly and the other on your chest.

   As you exhale through the nose, gently contract your abdominal muscles and push all of the air out of your belly and lungs. The hand on your belly should move inwards. Think of moving your belly towards the back of the chair.

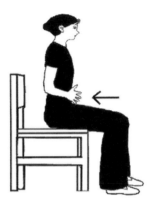

   As you inhale through the nose let the belly rise first. Your belly and the hand on your belly should move outwards with the inhalation. Then let the chest and the hand on the chest rise next. It may take some practice to have the belly move first, or at all. Do not let the shoulders rise up when inhaling. They should stay down and relaxed the entire time.

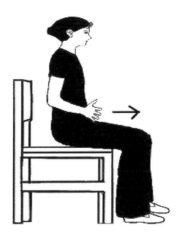

Rhythmic Limbering Exercises

Before beginning any exercise routine it is important to "warm-up" the body. "Warming-up" simply means preparing the joints and muscles for movement, and allowing the heart and breathing rate to increase slowly. The following exercises help loosen the joints and muscles and bring oxygen to the body, which can make the body more receptive to aerobic, strength training, and flexibility exercises. The following are some basic movements you can do to help prepare the body for aerobic exercise. The following exercises are shown both seated and standing. Do as much as you can standing to help get your balance before beginning the aerobic exercises.

Breathe and Reach

Before starting check your posture. Stand or sit up straight, bring the hips under the shoulders, and think about pushing the crown of the head up to the ceiling without lifting the chin. Arms are down by your sides.

Inhale bringing the arms up overhead and step the feet apart. Make sure the shoulders stay down. As you exhale lower the arms back to your sides. Repeat 3 times.

Standing

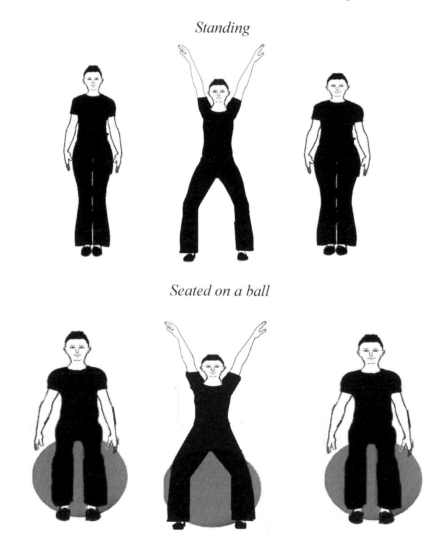

Seated on a ball

Squat and Reach Overhead

Before starting check your posture. Stand or sit up straight, bring the hips under the shoulders, and think about pushing the crown of the head up to the ceiling without lifting the chin.

Squat down only as far as you can without hurting your knees. Then stand up and reach the right arm overhead. Squat down again. Then stand up and reach the left arm overhead. Do 8-12 repetitions alternating right to left.

Standing

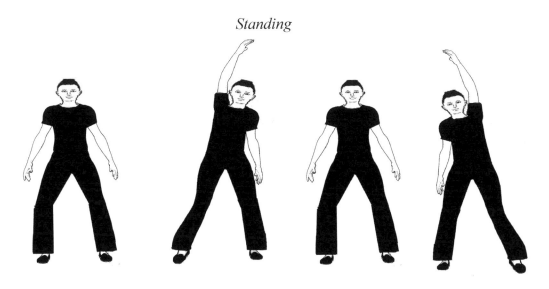

Seated on a ball

Gently bounce down and then reach your arm as you come up

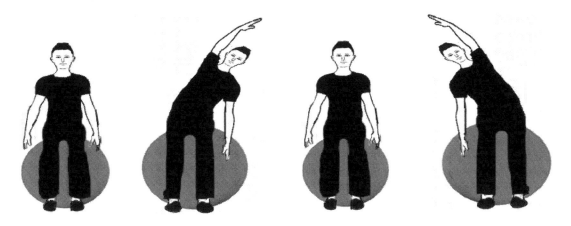

Checklist
- ✓ Stand or sit up straight. Think of pushing the crown of the head up to the ceiling without lifting the chin
- ✓ Do as much as you can standing without holding on
- ✓ Only squat as low as your knees comfortably allow
- ✓ Breathe

Squat and Reach Forward

Before starting check your posture. Stand or sit up straight, bring the hips under the shoulders, and think about pushing the crown of the head up to the ceiling without lifting the chin.

Squat down only as far as you can without hurting your knees. Then stand up and reach the right arm across the body chest height. Be careful to not twist the back or knees, keep the hips and shoulders facing forward. Squat down again. Then stand up and reach the left arm across the body chest height. Do 8-12 repetitions alternating right to left.

Standing

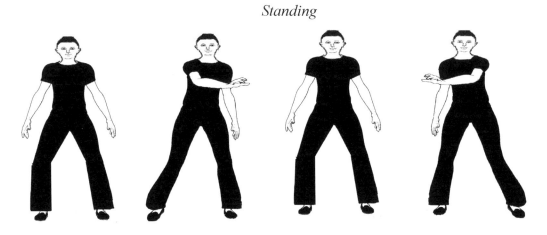

Seated on a ball
Gently bounce down and then reach your arm as you come up

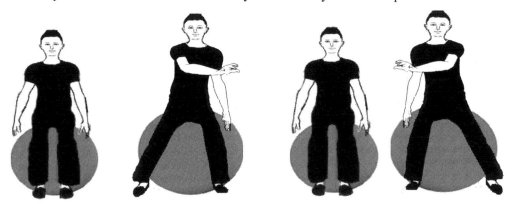

Checklist
✓ Stand or sit up straight. Think of pushing the crown of the head up to the ceiling without lifting the chin
✓ Do as much as you can standing without holding on
✓ Only squat as low as your knees comfortably allow
✓ Keep the hips and shoulders facing forward
✓ Do not twist the knees or back
✓ Breathe

Squat and Swing The Arms

Before starting check your posture. Stand or sit up straight, bring the hips under the shoulders, and think about pushing the crown of the head up to the ceiling without lifting the chin.

Squat down only as far as you can without hurting your knees. Then stand up and swing both arms across the body to the right. Be careful to not twist the back or knees. Squat down again. Then stand up and swing both arms across the body to the left. Do 8-12 repetitions alternating right to left.

Standing

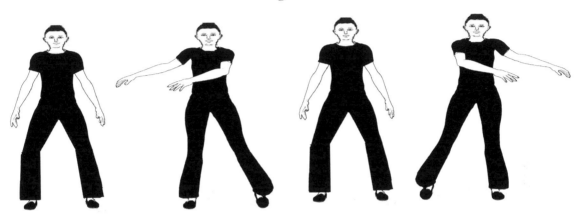

Seated on a ball
Gently bounce down and then swing your arm as you come up

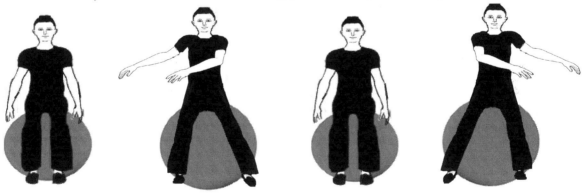

Checklist
- ✓ Stand or sit up straight. Think of pushing the crown of the head up to the ceiling without lifting the chin
- ✓ Do as much as you can standing without holding on
- ✓ Only squat as low as your knees comfortably allow
- ✓ Do not twist the back or the knees
- ✓ Breathe

55

Heel To Toe Rock

Before starting check your posture. Stand or sit up straight, bring the hips under the shoulders, and think about pushing the crown of the head up to the ceiling without lifting the chin.

Rock forward tapping the back toe on the floor and lift the arms up to the front. Then rock back tapping the front heel and swing the arms back. Continue back and forth 8-12 times. Repeat other side.

Standing

Tap back toes   *Tap front heel*

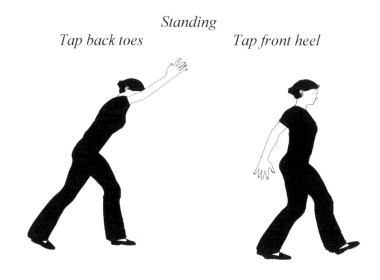

Seated on a ball

Alternate between lifting the toes and then the heels.

Lift Toes   *Lift Heels*

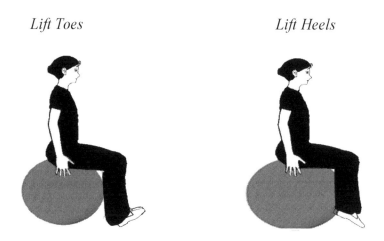

Checklist
- ✓ Stand or sit up straight. Think of pushing the crown of the head up to the ceiling without lifting the chin
- ✓ Do as much as you can standing without holding on
- ✓ Breathe

Hamstring Stretch

Before starting check your posture. Stand or sit up straight, bring the hips under the shoulders, and think about pushing the crown of the head up to the ceiling without lifting the chin.

Stand in a lunge position with the right leg forward and the left leg back. Make sure both the front toes and the back toes are pointing forward and do not turn the back leg out. Bend your front knee and press your back heel to the floor. Line the front knee over the front ankle and make sure the front knee does not go past the front ankle. You should be able to look down at your right knee and see your toes.

Hold for 5-10 deep breaths. Repeat on the other side. You can hold onto a chair or counter if needed to maintain balance and then try to work up to not holding on.

Standing

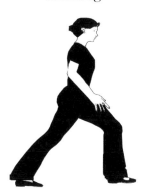

Seated on a ball

When seated make sure you keep the back straight. Come forward with your chest and do not round the back.

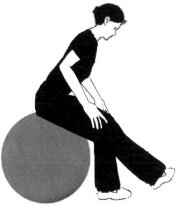

Checklist
- ✓ Stand or sit up straight. Think of pushing the crown of the head up to the ceiling without lifting the chin
- ✓ Do as much as you can standing without holding on
- ✓ When standing keep the front knee aligned over the front ankle
- ✓ When seated keep the back straight and lean forward with the chest
- ✓ Breathe

Quadriceps Stretch

Before starting check your posture. Stand or sit up straight, bring the hips under the shoulders, and think about pushing the crown of the head up to the ceiling without lifting the chin.

Stand in a lunge position with the right leg forward and the left leg back. Make sure both the front toes and the back toes are pointing forward and do not turn the back leg out. Drop your back knee down as far as you comfortably can. Line the front knee over the front ankle and make sure the front knee does not go past the front ankle. You should be able to look down at your right knee and see your toes.

Hold for 5-10 deep breaths. Repeat on the other side. You can hold onto a chair or counter if needed to maintain balance and then try to work up to not holding on.

Standing

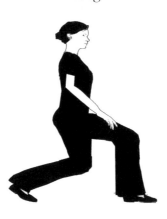

Seated on a ball
Reach the toes back and focus on pulling the hips under the shoulders.

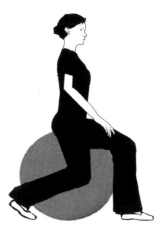

Checklist
✓ Stand or sit up straight. Think of pushing the crown of the head up to the ceiling without lifting the chin
✓ Do as much as you can standing without holding on
✓ Only go as low as you can without causing knee pain
✓ Keep the front knee aligned over the front ankle
✓ Breathe

58

Marching In Place

Alternately lift the feet off the floor and swing the arms.

Standing

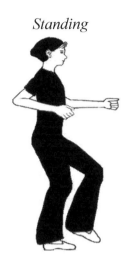

Standing with assistance

Do not lean on the chair or grab it too tightly; use a light fingertip grip. Let your legs work to support you.

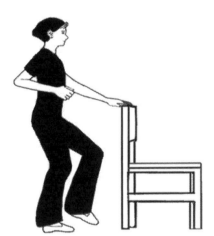

Seated on a ball or chair

You can also march in place while sitting on a chair or a ball.
Push down into the ball each time before you lift your foot – hold onto a chair if needed.

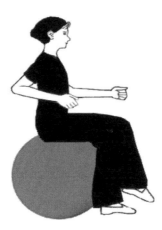

In the chair - sit up straight and away from the back of the chair as much as possible.

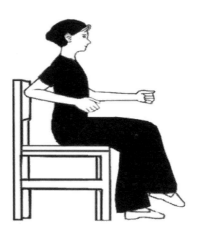

Checklist
✓ Stand or sit up straight. Think of pushing the crown of the head up to the ceiling without lifting the chin
✓ Do as much as you can standing without holding on
✓ Swing your arms, using opposite arm to leg
✓ Try to avoid swinging the same arm as leg, which can bring you out of balance
✓ Focus on picking up the fet so they come completely off the floor.
✓ Periodically use the Rating of Perceived Exertion or talk test (pg. 41) to check if you are exercising at the right level
✓ Breathe

Alternate Straight Leg Kicks

Alternately kick forward with a straight leg. Kick as high as you can keeping your balance and your back straight. Swing the opposite arm to leg.

Standing

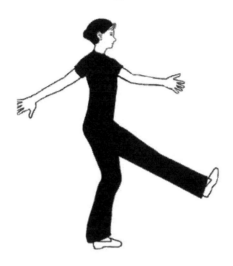

Standing with assistance

Do not lean on the chair or grab it too tightly; use a light fingertip grip. Let your legs work to support you.

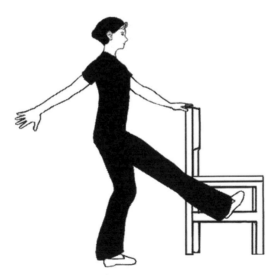

Seated on a ball or chair
You can also kick while sitting on a chair or a ball.
Push down into the ball each time before you lift your foot – hold onto a chair if needed.

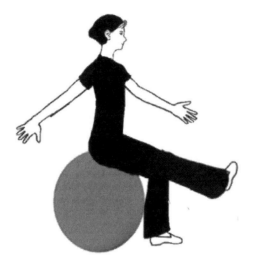

In the chair - sit up straight and away from the back of the chair as much as possible.

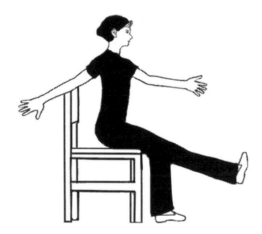

Checklist
- ✓ Stand or sit up straight. Think of pushing the crown of the head up to the ceiling without lifting the chin
- ✓ Do as much as you can standing without holding on
- ✓ Swing your arms, using opposite arm to leg
- ✓ Try to avoid swinging the same arm as leg, which can bring you out of balance
- ✓ Focus on keeping the knee straight
- ✓ Periodically use the Rating of Perceived Exertion or talk test (pg. 41) to check if you are exercising at the right level
- ✓ Breathe

Stepping Side to Side

Standing

Stand with feet together.   Step out to the right.   Bring the left foot to the right foot

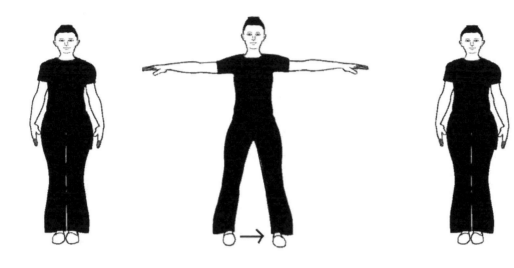

Stand with feet together.   Step out to the left.   Bring the right foot to the left foot

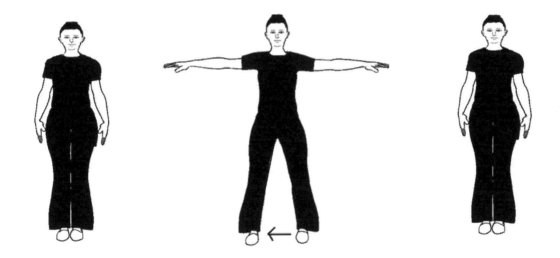

Continue stepping from right to left. Try to swing the arms up to shoulder height.

Standing with assistance

Do not lean on the chair or counter or grab it too tightly; use a light fingertip grip. Let your legs work to support you.

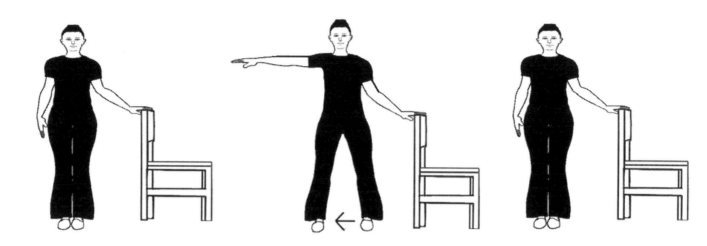

Continue stepping from side to side

Seated on chair

You can also step side to side while sitting in a chair

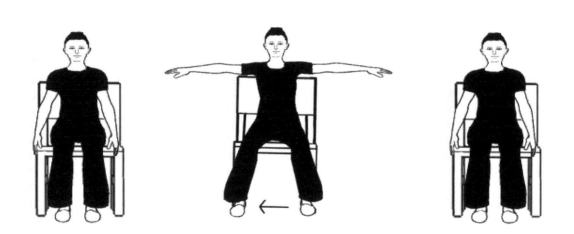

Jumping jacks on the ball

If sitting on a ball do jumping jacks instead of stepping side to side.

Push down into the ball. Then jump or step the feet apart. Swing the arms out to the side and up overhead if you can. Then jump or step the feet back together. Make sure you land on a flat foot and do not bounce on the toes as this can stress the shins. Push down into the ball as much as you can each time before you bring the legs apart. The more you push into the ball, the more aerobic the exercise becomes.

Push down

Bounce up and jump or step the feet apart
Hold onto a chair if needed for balance

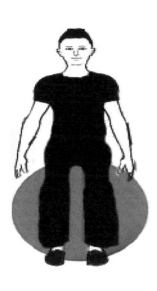

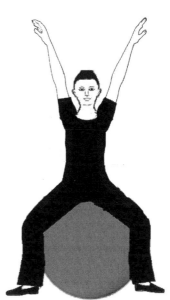

Checklist
✓ Stand or sit up straight. Think of pushing the crown of the head up to the ceiling without lifting the chin
✓ Do as much as you can standing without holding on
✓ Swing your arms up to shoulder height level
✓ Focus on taking as wide of a step as you can
✓ Periodically use the Rating of Perceived Exertion or talk test (pg. 41) to check if you are exercising at the right level
✓ Breathe

Alternate Knee Lifts

Alternately lift your knees as high as you can while keeping your balance and your back straight. Swing the opposite arm to leg.

Standing

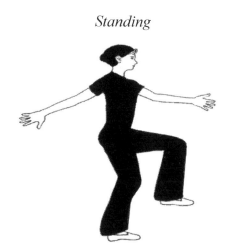

Standing with assistance

Do not lean on the chair or grab it too tightly; use a light fingertip grip. Let your legs work to support you.

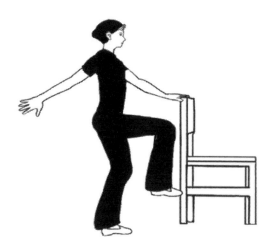

Seated on a ball or chair

You can also lift your knees while sitting on a chair or a ball.

Push down into the ball each time before you lift your foot – hold onto a chair if needed.

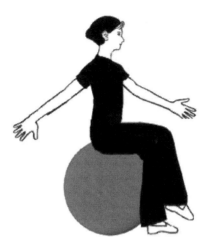

In the chair - sit up straight and away from the back of the chair as much as possible.

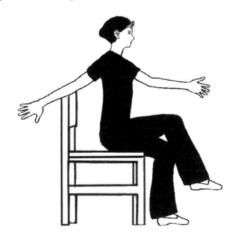

Checklist
- ✓ Stand or sit up straight. Think of pushing the crown of the head up to the ceiling without lifting the chin
- ✓ Do as much as you can standing without holding on
- ✓ Swing your arms, using opposite arm to leg
- ✓ Try to avoid swinging the same arm as leg, which can bring you out of balance
- ✓ Focus on bringing the knee up to waist height if you can
- ✓ Periodically use the Rating of Perceived Exertion or talk test (pg. 41) to check if you are exercising at the right level
- ✓ Breathe

Side Toe Tap

Reach the right toe directly out to the side, as the arms lift up to the side. Do not put any weight on the toe. Keep your weight in the left leg.
Bring the right leg back to the center.
Reach the left toe directly out to the side, as the arms lift up to the side. Do not put any weight on the toe. Keep your weight in the right leg.
Bring the left leg back to the center.
Continue alternating from side to side.

Standing

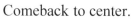

Tap the right toe to the side, reaching the arms out.

Comeback to center.

Tap the left toe to the side, reaching the arms out.

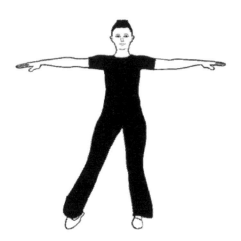
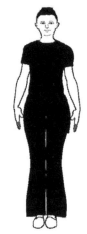
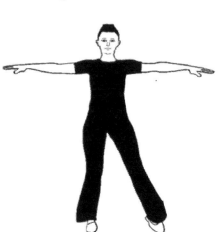

Standing with assistance

Do not lean on the chair or counter or grab it too tightly; use a light fingertip grip. Let your legs work to support you.

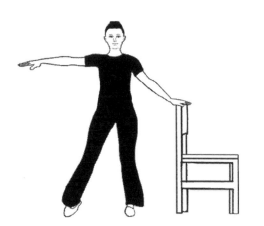
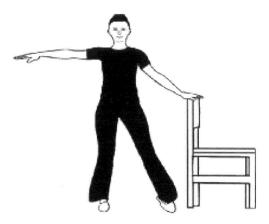

Seated on a ball or chair
You can also do side toe taps while sitting in a chair or on a ball.

*Bounce up and tap the toe
out to the side*

Push down in the center

*Bounce up and tap to the
other side*

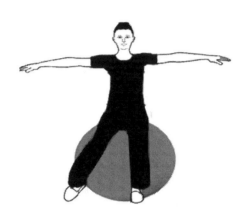 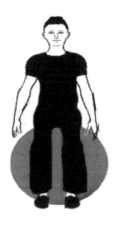 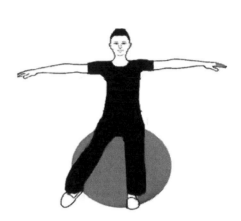

In the chair - sit up straight and away from the back of the chair as much as possible.

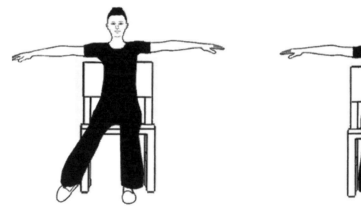 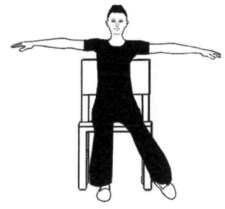

Checklist
- ✓ Stand or sit up straight. Think of pushing the crown of the head up to the ceiling without lifting the chin
- ✓ Do as much as you can standing without holding on
- ✓ Swing your arms and bring them shoulder height if possible
- ✓ Reach the toe directly out to the side as far as you can without putting any weight in the toe
- ✓ Face forward through this movement. Do not twist the back or knees
- ✓ Periodically use the Rating of Perceived Exertion or talk test (pg. 41) to check if you are exercising at the right level
- ✓ Breathe

Alternate Forward Heel Taps

Flex the foot and tap just the heel of the foot on the ground in front of you. Do not place the whole foot on the floor, or put any weight on the front foot. Alternately tap heels in front. Swing opposite arm to foot.

Standing

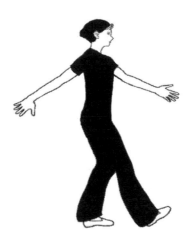

Standing with assistance

Do not lean on the chair or grab it too tightly; use a light fingertip grip. Let your legs work to support you.

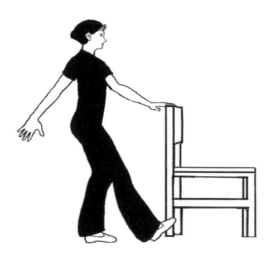

Seated on a ball or chair
You can also do heel taps while sitting on a chair or a ball.
Push down into the ball each time before you tap your heel – hold onto a chair if needed.

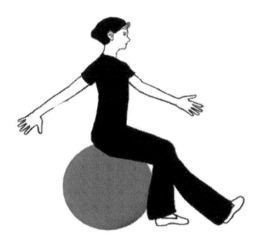

In the chair - sit up straight and away from the back of the chair as much as possible.

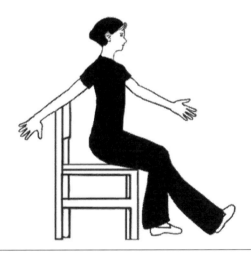

Checklist
- ✓ Stand or sit up straight. Think of pushing the crown of the head up to the ceiling without lifting the chin
- ✓ Do as much as you can standing without holding on
- ✓ Swing your arms, using opposite arm to leg
- ✓ Try to avoid swinging the same arm as leg, which can bring you out of balance
- ✓ Focus on touching just the heel on the floor and keeping your weight in your back leg
- ✓ Periodically use the Rating of Perceived Exertion or talk test (pg. 41) to check if you are exercising at the right level
- ✓ Breathe

Putting It All Together

Quick Reference List

Start with three to five minutes of rhythmic limbering exercises or a short walk.

1. March in Place.
2. Alternate Straight Leg Kicks.
3. Stepping Side to Side or Jumping Jacks on the ball.
4. Alternate Knee Lifts.
5. Side Toe Tap.
6. Alternate Forward Heel Taps.

The 3 1/2 Minute Workout.

1. March in Place …..................…. 35 seconds
2. Alternate Straight Leg Kicks .…. 35 seconds
3. Stepping Side to Side…............. 35 seconds
4. Alternate Knee Lifts................… 35 seconds
5. Side Toe Tap…......................... 35 seconds
6. Alternate Forward Heel Taps…. 35 seconds

The 7 Minute Workout.

1. March in Place …..................…. 70 seconds
2. Alternate Straight Leg Kicks …. 70 seconds
3. Stepping Side to Side…............. 70 seconds
4. Alternate Knee Lifts…............... 70 seconds
5. Side Toe Tap…......................... 70 seconds
6. Alternate Forward Heel Taps…. 70 seconds

The 10 Minute Workout.

1. March in Place …...................... 50 seconds
2. Alternate Straight Leg Kicks … 50 seconds
3. Stepping Side to Side…............. 50 seconds
4. Alternate Knee Lifts…............... 50 seconds
5. Side Toe Tap…........................ 50 seconds
6. Alternate Forward Heel Taps….50 seconds
7. March in Place …...................... .50 seconds
8. Alternate Straight Leg Kicks ….50 seconds
9. Stepping Side to Side…............. 50 seconds
10. Alternate Knee Lifts…............... .50 seconds
11. Side Toe Tap…........................ .50 seconds
12. Alternate Forward Heel Taps… 50 seconds

The 14 Minute Workout.

1. March in Place …...................... 70 seconds
2. Alternate Straight Leg Kicks …. 70 seconds
3. Stepping Side to Side…............. 70 seconds
4. Alternate Knee Lifts…................ 70 seconds
5. Side Toe Tap............................ 70 seconds
6. Alternate Forward Heel Taps…. 70 seconds
7. March in Place …...................... 70 seconds
8. Alternate Straight Leg Kicks …. 70 seconds
9. Stepping Side to Side….............. 70 seconds
10. Alternate Knee Lifts…................ 70 seconds
11. Side Toe Tap…........................ 70 seconds
12. Alternate Forward Heel Taps…. 70 seconds

Checklist
- ✓ Try creating your own sequence of movements to make up your aerobic workout
- ✓ Try moving around the room; march forward for 8, march back for 8, or when side stepping, travel 4 steps right then 4 steps left, etc.
- ✓ Remember the object is to keep moving, and to keep the heart rate up
- ✓ Try incorporating your favorite music into your routine
- ✓ Start slowly and build up gradually so your body can adapt
- ✓ Listen to your body to determine the appropriate level for each day
- ✓ Remember to use the Rating of Perceived Exertion or talk test (pg. 41) to check if you are exercising at the right level

Chapter Three

Strength Training

"Never be bullied into silence. Never allow yourself to be made a victim. Accept no one's definition of your life; define yourself."
- Harvey Fierstein

Strength training or resistance training is another important component of an exercise program for those with MS. As the muscles become stronger, certain tasks such as standing, walking, rising from a chair, climbing stairs, and lifting objects becomes easier. Strength training or resistance training simply means performing movements against some kind of resistance. Such resistance can be your own body weight, free weights such as hand and ankle weights, theraband or tubing, or machines typically found at gyms. When beginning a strength training routine, it is advisable to have the guidance of an instructor to make sure you are performing the movements correctly. Aside from this you can get a complete and beneficial strength training workout at home.

Benefits of strength training include:

➤ Stronger muscles that can do bigger jobs (such as lifting heavier objects)
➤ Stronger muscles that will work longer before becoming exhausted
➤ Increase in lean body mass (more muscle, less fat)
➤ Increase in metabolism meaning more calories burned even at rest
➤ Increase in bone mineral density (stronger bones)
➤ Improvements in overall stability and balance
➤ Lower blood sugar levels
➤ Decrease in body fat
➤ Fewer body aches and less fatigue

If you have access to hand and ankle weights, this book will show you how to use them. However, when beginning an exercise routine you should use light weights. You will find that you will be able to increase the weight fairly quickly in the beginning. Eventually you will find a weight which you will use for a while. If you do not have weights at home you can use common household items to start, and wait to buy weights when you are ready for more resistance. Instead of hand weights try using full soup cans or cylinder-shaped plastic containers filled with water or sand. Plastic shampoo, milk bottles, or laundry detergent containers work well. For ankle weights you can substitute with an old pair of socks filled with sand to the appropriate weight. These can and then be tied or fastened with Velcro around your ankles.

Most people in our classes start with three pound weights. We suggest only doing 8-12 repetitions of each exercise, so this weight should be good for most. Using less may not give you enough resistance to gain strength. Using less weight with more repetitions does not provide as effective results. One way to help determine the appropriate amount of weight to use is a technique known as the "10 Rep Max." This means finding the maximum amount of weight you can lift for 10 repetitions. For example, if you can lift three pounds more than 10 times with no difficulty and with good form, then that weight is too light for you. On the other hand if you can just about do 10 repetitions with good form with five pound weights before getting too tired to continue, than five pounds is a good weight for you to use. However if you are rehabilitating from an injury, check with your healthcare provider to determine if using weights is appropriate for your situation. *Never* sacrifice good lifting technique or range of motion for weight. If the weight is too heavy to allow you to do the exercise correctly through the full range of motion, do not use weight or switch to a lighter weight. If you cannot perform the full range of motion even without weight, check with your healthcare provider about seeing a physical or occupational therapist who can address the issue. It is essential for those with MS to do all they can to maintain as much range of motion in the joints as possible in order to remain active.

Some tips to make your strength training routine safe and effective follow.

➢ Stop any exercise that causes pain.
➢ Perform all of the movements *slowly and with control*. Use a *"four thousand count"* for each exercise to both lift and lower the weight.
➢ Practice good posture and body mechanics while doing the exercises.
➢ Exhale when lifting the weight and inhale while lowering the weight.
➢ Do not grip hand weights too tightly. This can cause a rise in blood pressure.
➢ Movements should be done with precision. Do not use rapid or "jerky" movements, and *never* just swing the weights or body through the movements.
➢ Do not perform strengthening exercises on the same muscles two days in a row. Your muscles need 48 hours after lifting to repair and recover. If you need or wish to split up your routine, try working your arms one day, and your legs the next, but you should not work the same muscles on two consecutive days.
➢ Perform 8-12 repetitions of each exercise.
➢ When you are able to perform 12 repetitions with no difficulty and with good form, increase the amount of weight by two to three pounds.
➢ If you are unable to perform the entire series of strengthening exercises at one time, you can split the routine doing certain exercises at different times throughout the day, or by working your legs one day and your arms the next day.
➢ You may find you need different weights for different exercises, i.e., five pound weights for larger muscles and three pound weights for the smaller muscles.
➢ *Always "warm-up" before lifting weights to avoid injury.*

The leg exercises will be illustrated in both standing and seated positions. Do as much as you can standing. When standing, it is strongly recommended that you hold onto a chair or counter for support. For this section it is important to challenge yourself with the weight or resistance. By holding on you lessen your chances of a fall allowing you to fully focus on lifting the weight. The upper body exercises will be illustrated in a seated position. This again reduces the risk for a fall, enabling you to focus on challenging yourself with weight. Also, when performing upper body exercises, it is sometimes easier to maintain a straight back while seated. Lifting weights while standing, especially with heavier weights, can often lead to arching the back or locking the knees in order to lift the weight. Accompanying each exercise is a diagram highlighting the muscle or muscle group the exercise is targeting. Although most exercises utilize additional muscles that assist and stabilize movement, the diagrams highlight the primary muscle or muscle group each exercise is targeting. In general, when strength training, it is usually recommended to start with the largest muscles in your body first; i.e., your legs, and work down to the smaller muscles in your arms. However, if are working with some type of split routine or altering the workout, do what works best for you.

Remember to proceed slowly and use correct form. With all movements in this book, use your own judgment as to what is right for your body each day.

Strength Training Exercises

Leg Extension   *Muscles worked: Quadriceps (Front top of thigh)*
(Rectus femoris, vastus lateralis, vastus medialis, and vastus intermedius).

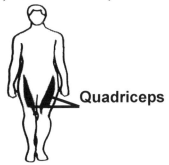

Standing

Before starting, check your posture. Stand up straight, bring the hips under the shoulders, and think about pushing the crown of the head to the ceiling without lifting the chin. Do 8-12 repetitions with the right leg, then 8-12 repetitions with the left leg.

Stand straight.	Lift the knee.	Straighten the leg.

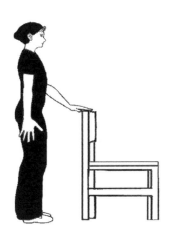 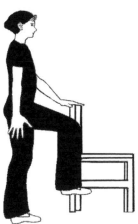 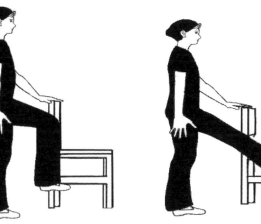

Bend the knee.	Put the foot down.

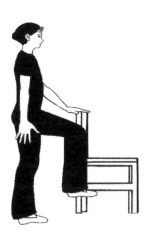 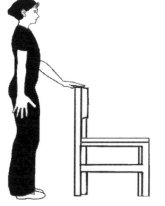

Seated

Sit up straight, away from the back of the chair if possible. If you need to sit back, sit all the way back to avoid slouching.

Sit up straight.　　　Lift the knee.　　　Straighten the leg.

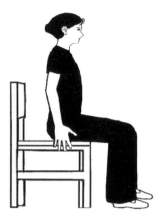 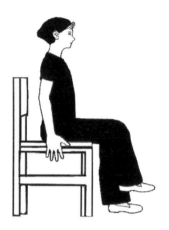 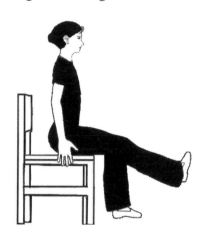

Bend the knee.　　　Put the foot down.

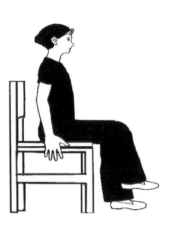 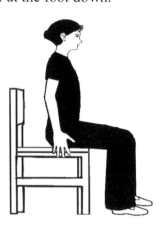

Checklist
- ✓ Stand or sit up straight
- ✓ If possible do all repetitions on one leg and then switch to the other leg. If this bothers your hips or back you can alternate legs
- ✓ Move through your full range of motion, but do not lock the knee
- ✓ Ankle weights may be used if that feels appropriate
- ✓ Exhale as you lift the leg, inhale as you lower the leg
- ✓ Move slowly using a 4 thousand count both to lift the leg and to lower the leg
- ✓ Use diaphragmatic breathing through the nose as much as possible
- ✓ Do not exercise to the point of strain or discomfort

Wall Slides *Muscles worked: Quadriceps (Front top of thigh)*
(Rectus femoris, vastus lateralis, vastus medialis, and vastus intermedius).

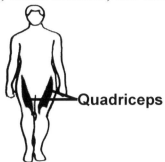

Place the physioball against the wall at low back height. Stand a few feet away from the ball and lean back until your low back is pressing into the ball. Begin to bend your knees and slide down no lower than a 45-degree angle and hold. The ball will roll up to your upper back. Keep your heels on the floor and press into your heels to come back up. Make sure you do not lock the knees when you come back up to standing. Repeat 8-12 times.

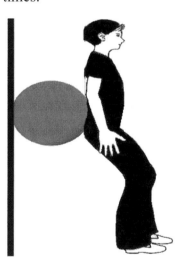 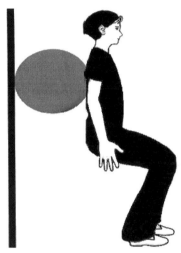

Checklist
- ✓ Stand away from the wall so you are leaning against the ball
- ✓ Move slowly using a 4 thousand count to go down and when coming up
- ✓ Only go as low as you can without causing knee pain
- ✓ Use diaphragmatic breathing through the nose as much as possible
- ✓ Keep the knees slightly bent when standing
- ✓ Keep the natural arch in the low back
- ✓ Do not exercise to the point of strain or discomfort

Side Leg Lift   *Muscles worked: Abductors (Hip, outer thigh)*
(Tensor fasciae late, gluteus medius, and gluteus minimus)

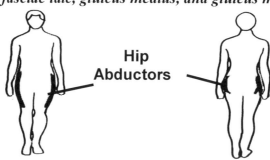

Standing

Before starting, check your posture. Stand up straight, bring the hips under the shoulders, and think about pushing the crown of the head to the ceiling without lifting the chin.

Turn your right foot in and lift the right leg straight out to the side as high as you can without tipping your body. Then lower slowly down. Do 8-12 repetitions with the right leg, then 8-12 repetitions with the left leg. Let the heel lead with the toes facing inward. *Do not let the leg turn out.*

Right

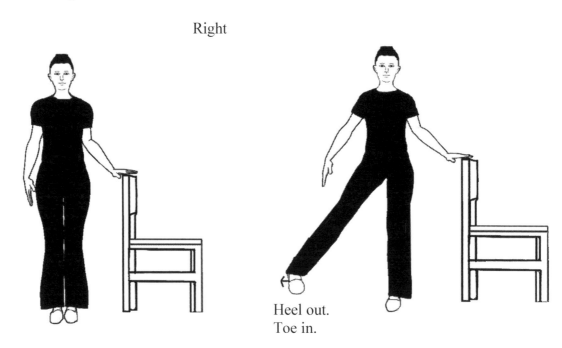

Heel out.
Toe in.

Left

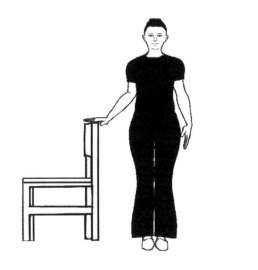 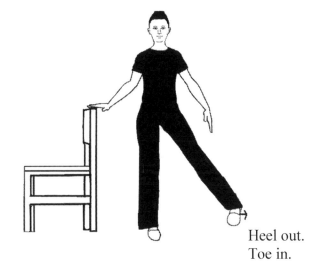

Heel out.
Toe in.

Seated

Sit up straight, away from the back of the chair if possible. If you need to sit back, sit all the way back to avoid slouching. Bring the leg out to the side without swinging the hips.

Right   Left

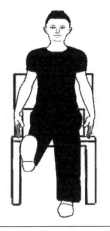 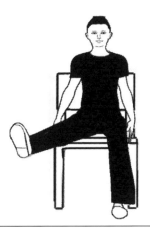 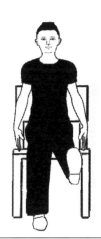 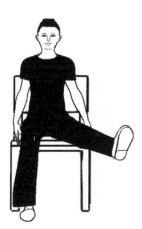

Checklist
- ✓ Stand or sit up straight
- ✓ If possible do all repetitions on one leg and then switch to the other leg. If this bothers your hips or back you can alternate legs
- ✓ Move through your full range of motion, but do not swing the hips
- ✓ Ankle weights may be used if that feels appropriate
- ✓ Exhale as you lift the leg, inhale as you lower the leg
- ✓ Move slowly using a 4 thousand count both to lift the leg and to lower the leg
- ✓ Use diaphragmatic breathing through the nose as much as possible
- ✓ Do not exercise to the point of strain or discomfort

Muscles worked: Gluteal & Hamstring Muscles (Buttocks, back top of thigh)
(Gluteus maximus, biceps femoris, semitendinosus, and semimembranosus)

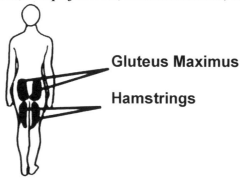

Before starting, check your posture. Stand up straight, bring the hips under the shoulders, and think about pushing the crown of the head to the ceiling without lifting the chin.

Standing Leg Lift Back

Stand straight. Tighten the buttocks muscles and flex your right foot. Lift the leg directly out to the back. Do not let the leg go out to the side. Do not let the shoulders tip forward. Then lower slowly down, Do 8-12 repetitions with the right leg, then 8-12 repetitions with the left leg.

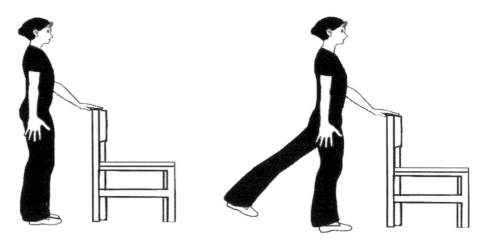

Seated Heel Curl

Sit up straight, away from the back of the chair if possible. If you need to sit back, sit all the way back to avoid slouching. Tighten the muscles in the back top of your thigh and squeeze the heel under the chair, or if your knee is sensitive bring the foot to the outside of the chair. Then return forward slowly. Do 8 – 12 repetitions with both legs.

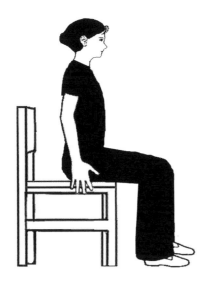 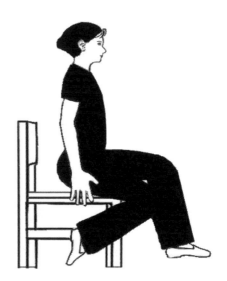

Checklist
✓ Stand or sit up straight. Do not let the shoulders tip forward
✓ If possible do all repetitions on one leg and then switch to the other leg. If this bothers your hips or back you can alternate legs
✓ Ankle weights may be used if that feels appropriate
✓ Exhale as you bring the leg back, inhale as you bring the leg forward
✓ Move slowly using a 4 thousand count both to lift the leg and to lower the leg
✓ Use diaphragmatic breathing through the nose as much as possible
✓ Do not exercise to the point of strain or discomfort

Leg Crossover   *Muscles worked: Adductor Muscles (Inner thigh)*
(Adductor longus, adductor brevis, and adductor magnus)

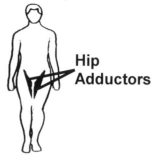

Standing

Before starting, check your posture. Stand up straight, bring the hips under the shoulders, and think about pushing the crown of the head to the ceiling without lifting the chin. Bring your leg across your body. Let the knee bend and think about lifting your heel up. Do 8-12 repetitions with the right leg, then 8-12 repetitions with the left leg.

Right

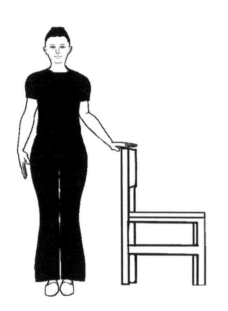 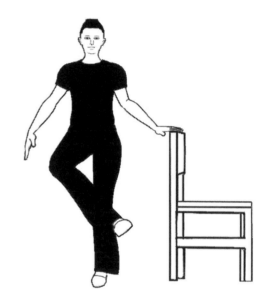

Left

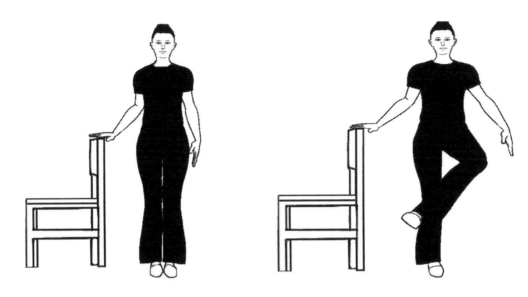

Seated

Sit up straight, away from the back of the chair if possible. If you need to sit back, sit all the way back to avoid slouching. Let the knee bend and drop out to the side and think about lifting your heel up. Then lower slowly down. Do eight to twelve repetitions on the right and then repeat with the left leg.

Right Leg   *Left Leg*

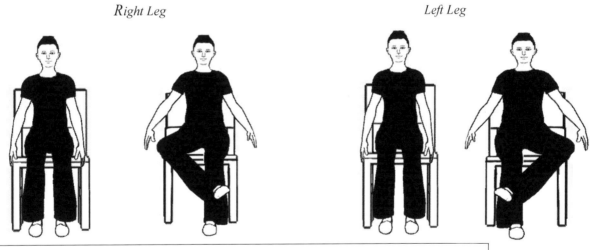

Checklist

- ✓ Stand or sit up straight
- ✓ If possible do all repetitions on one leg and then switch to the other leg. If this bothers your hips or back you can alternate legs
- ✓ Ankle weights may be used if that feels appropriate
- ✓ Exhale as you lift the leg, inhale as you lower the leg
- ✓ Move slowly using a 4 thousand count both to lift the leg and to lower the leg
- ✓ Use diaphragmatic breathing through the nose as much as possible
- ✓ Do not exercise to the point of strain or discomfort

Heel Raises   *Muscles worked: Gastrocnemius and Soleus (Calf)*
(Gastrocnemeus when standing and Soleus when seated)

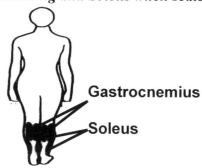

Standing

Before starting, check your posture. Stand up straight, bring the hips under the shoulders, and think about pushing the crown of the head to the ceiling without lifting the chin. Using the chair as little as possible, rise up onto the toes. When lowering just barely touch the heels, keeping most of the weight in the toes. Do 8-12 repetitions.

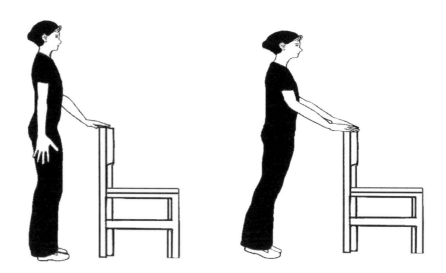

Seated

Sit up straight, away from the back of the chair if possible. If you need to sit back, sit all the way back to avoid slouching.

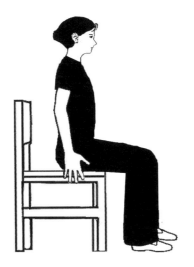 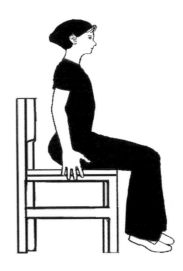

Checklist

✓ Stand or sit up straight
✓ Ankle weights may be used if that feels appropriate
✓ Try to keep the weight in your toes and not back in your heels
✓ Move slowly using a 4 thousand count both to lift the heels and to lower the heels
✓ Use diaphragmatic breathing through the nose as much as possible
✓ Do not exercise to the point of strain or discomfort

Toe Lifts
Muscles worked: Tibialis Anterior (Shin)

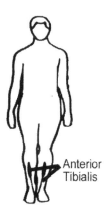

Standing

  Before starting, check your posture. Stand up straight, bring the hips under the shoulders, and think about pushing the crown of the head to the ceiling without lifting the chin. Using the chair as little as possible, bend the knees slightly and lift up just the toes. Then lower slowly down. Make sure you do not rock the hips backwards and keep the heels down. Do eight to twelve repetitions.

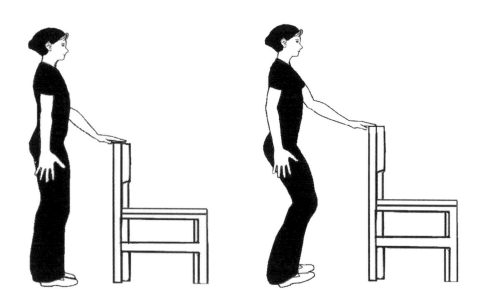

Seated

Sit up straight, away from the back of the chair if possible. If you need to sit back, sit all the way back to avoid slouching. Lift up the toes, keeping the heels down. Then lower slowly down. Make sure you do not rock the hips backwards and keep the heels down. Do eight to twelve repetitions.

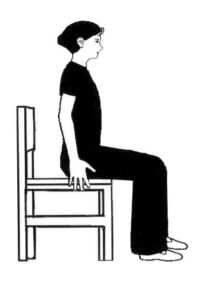 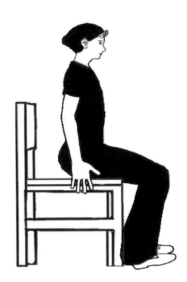

Checklist
- ✓ Stand or sit up straight
- ✓ Ankle weights may be used if that feels appropriate
- ✓ Avoid rocking back as you lift the toes
- ✓ Move slowly using a 4 thousand count both to lift the heels and to lower the heels
- ✓ Use diaphragmatic breathing through the nose as much as possible
- ✓ Do not exercise to the point of strain or discomfort

Wall Pushups/Seated Chest Fly   *Muscles worked: Pectoralis Major (Chest)*

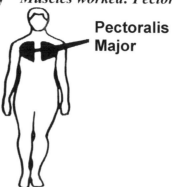

Pectoralis
Major

Before starting, check your posture. Stand or sit up straight, bring the hips under the shoulders, and think about pushing the crown of the head to the ceiling without lifting the chin.

Stand arms-length away from the wall. Place your hands chest height and shoulder width apart. Bend the elbows and bring your nose and chest as close to the wall as possible, keeping your hips and shoulders in one line. Do not let your hips come forward. Then push back out until the elbows are straight but not locked. Do 8-12 repetitions.

Standing Wall Pushup

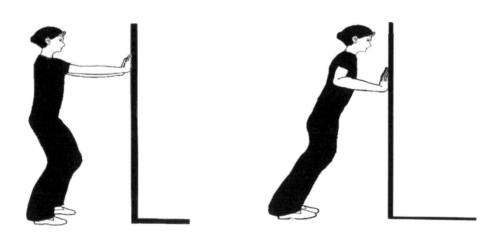

Seated Chest Fly

If you prefer to work seated you can isolate the same muscles with the seated chest fly. Sit at the very front edge of the chair. Then lean back so your upper back touches the chair for support. Do not drop your head back – keep your neck straight and in alignment.

Keeping the elbows slightly bent, open your arms out to the side. Do not let the wrists, hands or weights drop, make sure you control the movement. Then bring the weights up in front of your chest (not your face) in a circular motion – like you were hugging something. Keep your elbows bent throughout this movement – both when opening the arms and lifting the arms. Exhale as you lift the weights, inhale as you lower them. Do eight to twelve repetitions.

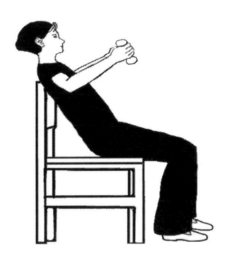 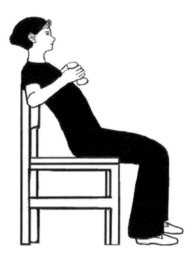

Checklist
- ✓ If standing, stand up straight
- ✓ Do not lock the elbows
- ✓ Keep your body straight, do not let the hips and buttocks come forward
- ✓ Move slowly using a 4 thousand count to both push away from the wall and as you lower yourself towards the wall
- ✓ Exhale as you push away from the wall, inhale as you come to the wall
- ✓ Use diaphragmatic breathing through the nose as much as possible
- ✓ Do not exercise to the point of strain or discomfort

Muscles worked: Trapezius, Rhomboids, Latissimus Dorsi (Upper and mid back)

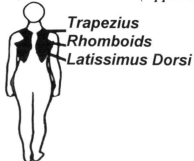

This exercise can be done seated or standing. The seated version may isolate the muscles better but it can place some strain on the back. Try both variations to see which version works best for you.

Standing

In standing, this exercise is illustrated using just one arm at a time, to better isolate the muscles and to protect the back. Stand in a lunge position and place your left hand on the chair for support. Keep your arm and elbow close to your body and squeeze the shoulder blades together as you lift the right elbow until your hand comes about waist height. Keep the abdominal muscles pulled in to protect the back. Do 8-12 repetitions with the right arm, then 8-12 repetitions with the left arm.

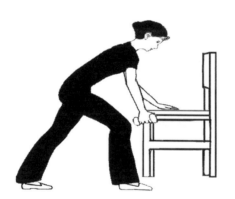 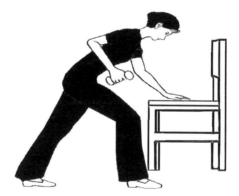

Seated

For the seated version, lean forward from the hips and look down and slightly ahead. Do not lift the head and compress the neck. Tighten the abdominal muscles and squeeze the shoulder blades together as you lift both elbows up until your hands come about waist height. Do 8-12 repetitions.

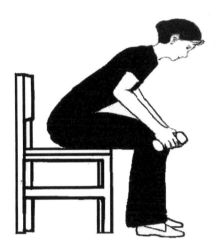 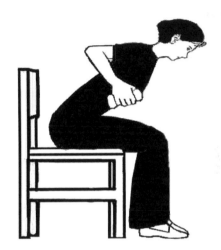

Checklist
- ✓ Keep the abdominal muscles in and the back straight
- ✓ Do not lock the elbows
- ✓ Hand weights may be used if that feels appropriate
- ✓ Move slowly using a 4 thousand count both to lift the weight and to lower the weight
- ✓ Exhale as you lift the weight up, inhale as you lower the weight down
- ✓ Use diaphragmatic breathing through the nose as much as possible
- ✓ Do not exercise to the point of strain or discomfort

Front Lateral Raise   *Muscles worked: Deltoid (Shoulders)*

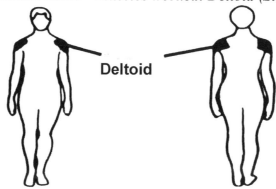

Deltoid

Before starting, check your posture. Sit at the front edge of the chair as much as possible in order to engage your abdominal muscles. If you need to sit back, sit all the way back in the chair to avoid slouching. Let the arms hang down at your sides with the palms facing back. Without rocking the body backwards lift the weights up in front of you to *shoulder height only*. If lifting both arms at the same time bothers your back you can do just one arm at a time. Do 8-12 repetitions.

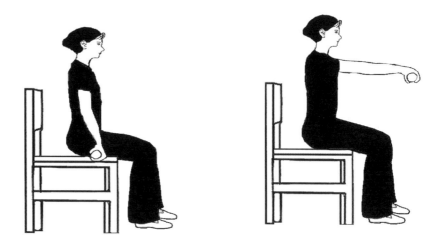

Checklist
- ✓ Sit up straight, away from the back of the chair if possible
- ✓ Hand weights may be used if that feels appropriate
- ✓ Exhale as you lift the weight up, inhale as you lower the weight
- ✓ Do not arch your back or rock backwards while lifting the weight
- ✓ Do not lock the elbows
- ✓ Make sure you only lift the weight to shoulder height
- ✓ Move slowly using a 4 thousand count both to lift the weight and to lower the weight
- ✓ Use diaphragmatic breathing through the nose as much as possible
- ✓ Do not exercise to the point of strain or discomfort

Military Press *Muscles worked: Deltoid and Trapezius (Shoulders)*

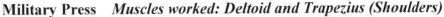
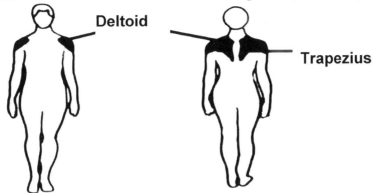

Deltoid

Trapezius

Before starting, check your posture. Sit at the front edge of the chair as much as possible in order to engage your abdominal muscles. If you need to sit back, sit all the way back in the chair to avoid slouching.

Bring your hands to shoulder height. Turn your palms so they face forward instead of facing your ears as this helps to open the shoulders and prevent forward rounding of the shoulders. Bring the arms back towards the ears as much as possible. Exhale as you lift the weights straight up overhead. Try to straighten your elbows without locking them. Then lower down just to shoulder height. Do 8-12 repetitions.

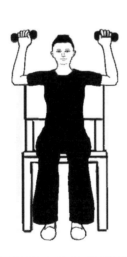
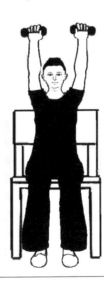

Checklist
- ✓ Sit up straight, away from the back of the chair if possible
- ✓ Hand weights may be used if that feels appropriate
- ✓ Exhale as you lift the weight up, inhale as you lower the weight
- ✓ Do not arch your back or rock backwards while lifting the weight
- ✓ Do not lock the elbows
- ✓ Turn the hands so the palms face forward to avoid rounding the shoulders forward
- ✓ Move slowly using a 4 thousand count both to lift the weight and to lower the weight
- ✓ Use diaphragmatic breathing through the nose as much as possible
- ✓ Do not exercise to the point of strain or discomfort

Deltoid Raise *Muscles worked: Deltoid (Shoulders)*

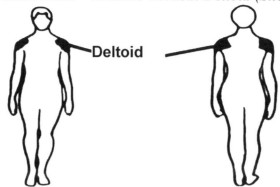

Deltoid

Before starting, check your posture. Sit at the front edge of the chair as much as possible in order to engage your abdominal muscles. If you need to sit back, sit all the way back in the chair to avoid slouching.

Bring your hands down by your side. Exhale as you lift straight up to the side, to shoulder height only. Your palms should be facing the floor. Keep your elbows straight but do not lock them. Do 8-12 repetitions.

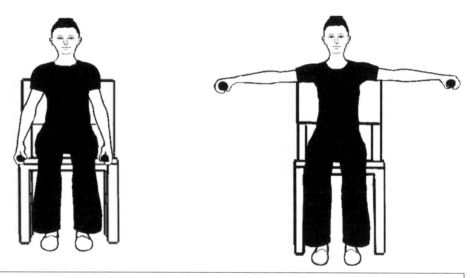

Checklist
- ✓ Sit up straight, away from the back of the chair if possible
- ✓ Hand weights may be used if that feels appropriate
- ✓ Exhale as you lift the weight up, inhale as you lower the weight
- ✓ Do not arch your back or rock backwards while lifting the weight
- ✓ Do not lock your elbows
- ✓ Move slowly using a 4 thousand count both to lift the weight and to lower the weight
- ✓ Use diaphragmatic breathing through the nose as much as possible
- ✓ Do not exercise to the point of strain or discomfort

Biceps Curl   *Muscles worked: Biceps (Front top of arm)*

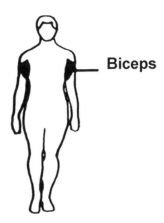

Biceps

Before starting, check your posture. Sit at the front edge of the chair as much as possible in order to engage your abdominal muscles. If you need to sit back, sit all the way back in the chair to avoid slouching.

Bring your hands down by your side. Turn your palms so they face forward. Exhale as you bend your elbows, bringing the weights to your shoulders. Keep your elbows at your side. Do not lift the elbows to bring the weight up. Do 8-12 repetitions.

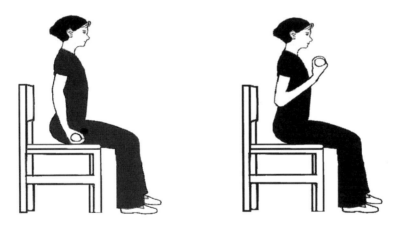

Checklist
- ✓ Sit up straight, away from the back of the chair if possible
- ✓ Hand weights may be used if that feels appropriate
- ✓ Exhale as you lift the weight up, inhale as you lower the weight
- ✓ Do not arch your back or rock backwards while lifting the weight
- ✓ Do not lock your elbows
- ✓ Move slowly using a 4 thousand count both to lift the weight and to lower the weight
- ✓ Use diaphragmatic breathing through the nose as much as possible
- ✓ Do not exercise to the point of strain or discomfort

Triceps Kickback   *Muscles worked: Triceps (Back top of arm)*

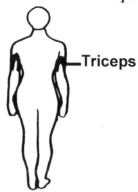

Before starting, check your posture. Sit at the front edge of the chair and tighten your abdominal muscles.

Bring your elbows into your side and lean slightly forward without straining your back. Leaning forward helps to better isolate the muscle. Keep the abdominal muscles tight. Straighten your arms and bring the weights back. Then, just bend at the elbow to bring the hand back. Avoid swinging the whole arm. The movement is just at the elbow joint. If doing both arms at the same time bothers your back you can do just one arm at a time. Do 8-12 repetitions.

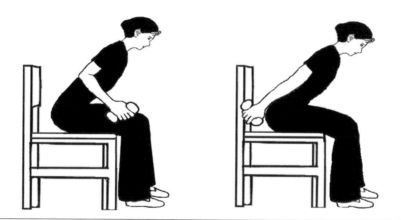

Checklist
✓ Lean forward enough to better isolate the muscle, but not too far as to strain the back
✓ Hand weights may be used if that feels appropriate
✓ Exhale as you straighten the elbow, inhale as you bend the elbow
✓ Do not arch your back or rock backwards while lifting the weight
✓ Do not lock your elbows
✓ Move slowly using a 4 thousand count both to straighten the elbow and to bend the elbow
✓ Use diaphragmatic breathing through the nose as much as possible
✓ Do not exercise to the point of strain or discomfort

Wrist Curls *Muscles worked: Flexor Carpi Radialis, Flexor Carpi Ulnaris*
(Front of wrists and forearm)

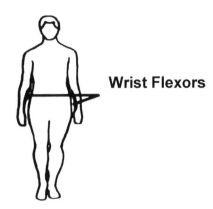

Wrist Flexors

Before starting, check your posture. Sit at the front edge of the chair as much as possible in order to engage your abdominal muscles. If you need to sit back, sit all the way back in the chair to avoid slouching.

Lean forward placing the back of your wrists and elbows on your thighs. Your hands should be past your knee. Hold the weight with the palms facing the ceiling. Exhale as you curl the wrist up. Keep the movement in the wrist only, do not lift your arms off of your thighs. Do 8-12 repetitions.

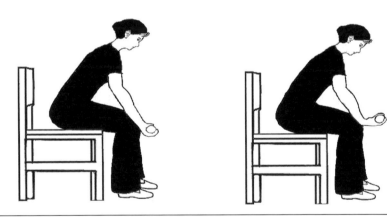

Checklist
✓ Sit up straight, away from the back of the chair if possible
✓ Hand weights may be used if that feels appropriate
✓ Exhale as you lift the weight up, inhale as you lower the weight
✓ Do not arch your back or rock backwards while lifting the weight
✓ Do not lift your elbow or forearm off of your thigh, keep the movement just in the wrist
✓ Move slowly using a 4 thousand count both to curl the wrist up and to lower the wrist
✓ Use diaphragmatic breathing through the nose as much as possible
✓ Do not exercise to the point of strain or discomfort

Reverse Wrist Curls

Muscles worked: Extensor Carpi Radialis Brevis, Extensor Carpi Ulnaris
(Back of wrists)

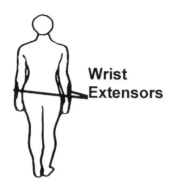

Wrist Extensors

Before starting, check your posture. Sit at the front edge of the chair as much as possible in order to engage your abdominal muscles. If you need to sit back, sit all the way back in the chair to avoid slouching.

Lean forward placing the front of your wrists and elbows on your thighs. Your hands should be past your knee. Hold the weight with the palms facing the floor. Exhale as you curl the wrist up. Keep the movement in the wrist only, do not lift your arms off of your thighs. Do 8-12 repetitions.

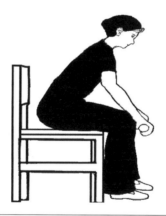 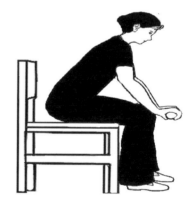

Checklist
✓ Sit up straight, away from the back of the chair if possible
✓ Hand weights may be used if that feels appropriate
✓ Exhale as you lift the weight up, inhale as you lower the weight
✓ Do not arch your back or rock backwards while lifting the weight
✓ Do not lift your elbow or forearm off of your thigh, keep the movement just in the wrist
✓ Move slowly using a 4 thousand count both to curl the wrist up and to lower the wrist
✓ Use diaphragmatic breathing through the nose as much as possible
✓ Do not exercise to the point of strain or discomfort

The last few exercises in the strength training segment can be done seated or on the floor. These exercises target your core muscles - the abdominals and obliques.

Lean Backs/Bicycles Seated *Muscles worked: Rectus Abdominus (Abdominal muscles)*

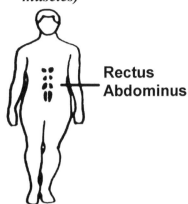

Rectus Abdominus

Before starting, check your posture. For this exercise you need to sit at the front edge of the chair so you have plenty of room to lean back.

Cross your arms at your chest. Inhale as you sit up straight letting the low back arch slightly. Exhale and tuck the chin into the chest. Let the low back round slightly and lean back. Go back far enough that you feel a pull in the abdominal muscles, but not so far that you touch the back of the chair. Make sure the back stays rounded. If you do not feel this exercise in your abdominal muscles you may be arching your back. Keep the chin tucked, do not let your head drop back. Keep the shoulders down and relaxed. Hold back for a five-second count, make sure you do not hold your breath. Inhale and come back up straight. Do 8-12 repetitions.

Sit up, low back arched slightly.   Lean back, chin tucked, back rounded.

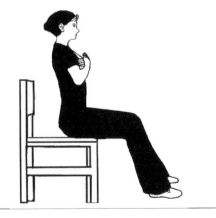
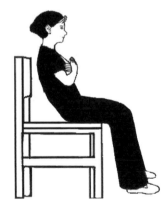

Checklist
- ✓ Sit up straight, away from the back of the chair if possible
- ✓ Inhale as you sit up, exhale as you lean back
- ✓ Keep the spine slightly rounded
- ✓ Do not drop the head back, keep the chin tucked
- ✓ Move slowly using a 4 thousand count both to lean back and to come forward
- ✓ Use diaphragmatic breathing through the nose as much as possible
- ✓ Do not exercise to the point of strain or discomfort

101

Bicycles
Lean back and bicycle both legs about 5 to 6 times.
Repeat for 6 to 8 repetitions.
This is a more challenging variation.
Remember to keep the abdominal muscles pulled in.

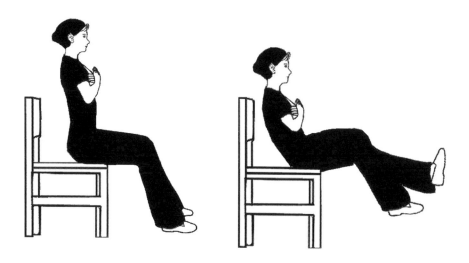

Checklist
✓ Inhale as you sit up, exhale as you lean back
✓ Keep the spine slightly rounded
✓ Do not drop the head back, keep the chin tucked
✓ Move slowly using a 4 thousand count both to lean back and to come forward
✓ Use diaphragmatic breathing through the nose as much as possible
✓ Do not exercise to the point of strain or discomfort

Side Bends *Muscles worked: Obliques (Waist)*

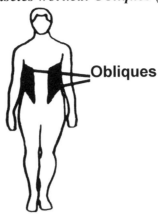

Obliques

Before starting, check your posture. Sit at the front edge of the chair as much as possible in order to engage your abdominal muscles. Inhale as you sit up straight. Exhale and bend to the right as far as you can. Do not lean forward, keep the shoulders over the hips. The elbows stay straight. As you come back up, let the waist muscles lift you up, and do not lift the weight with the arm. Keep the shoulders down and relaxed. Do 8-12 repetitions on the right, then 8-12 repetitions on the left.

Right   *Left*

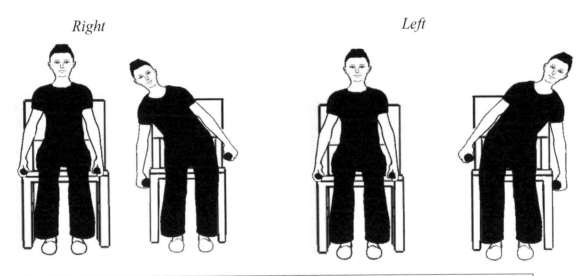

Checklist
✓ Sit up straight, away from the back of the chair if possible
✓ Inhale as you sit up, exhale as you bend
✓ Keep the spine straight and the shoulders over the hips
✓ Do not bend the elbows or lift the weights when sitting up. The movement is all in the waist
✓ Move slowly using a 4 thousand count both to bend to the side and to sit up straight
✓ Use diaphragmatic breathing through the nose as much as possible
✓ Do not exercise to the point of strain or discomfort

Floor Exercises

On days when you feel able floor exercises can be very beneficial. The floor is a solid surface that provides feedback as to whether or not the back is straight and you do not have to worry about falling. Doing floor exercises also keeps you in the habit of getting up and down. You may find that you will be able to get up more easily after a fall if you have been practicing getting up from the floor. Please refer to pages 35 through 38 for instructions as to how to get up and down safely. Performing these exercises on a couch or bed is not as beneficial as these surfaces are often too soft and do not provide enough support, however as always listen to your body and do what is best for you.

When performing floor exercises it is essential to maintain a pelvic tilt in the back in order to protect the back from injury. Letting your back arch off the floor can lead to back strain. It is also very important to keep your neck straight and in correct alignment. Make sure that the head does not tip backwards in order for your head to touch. This can place a lot of strain on the neck. To prevent neck strain place a towel or pillow under the head so the neck remains straight. However, do not use too high of a pillow as that will push the head forward. It is best to have someone help you get set up the first time so they can see if your neck is straight and to help you decide how much cushioning you need under your head.

Incorrect. Head tipped back   *Incorrect. Too much support*
                                                  Head pushed forward

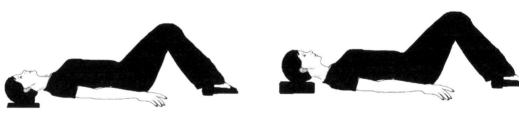

Correct Neck is straight and in alignment

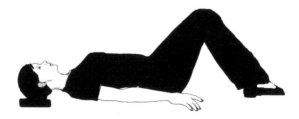

Pelvic Tilts

Lie on the floor on your back with the knees bent, feet on the floor. Make sure you keep the head and neck level, do not arch the head or tip the chin back. If you find that you are arching your neck, place a pillow under the head.

This exercise helps to strengthen the abdominal muscles and should be used with every floor exercise in order to protect the back from injury. Without lifting the hips or buttocks, press your low back down into the floor. Try to slip your hands under your low back. If you are doing this exercise correctly you should feel your low back tight against the floor, and you should be unable to get your hands under your back. Hold for a slow count of five. Then relax and let the low back arch enough so that you can slip your hands under your back. Repeat eight to twelve times.

Pelvic Tilt Down   *Pelvic Tilt Arch*

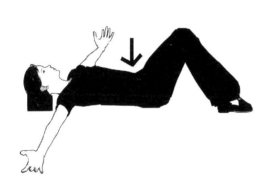
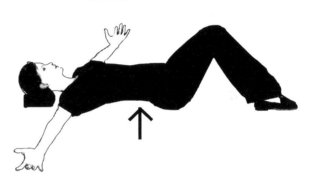

Checklist	
✓	Make sure you keep your head and chin level
✓	Make sure you are moving the just the low back and not lifting the hips or buttocks
✓	Use diaphragmatic breathing through the nose as much as possible
✓	Do not exercise to the point of strain or discomfort

Knee To Chest

This exercise strengthens the abdominal muscles. Lie on the floor on your back. Keep the head and neck level. If you find that you are arching your neck, place a pillow under the head. Begin with a pelvic tilt. Throughout this exercise make sure your low back stays in contact with the floor.

Without arching the back tighten your stomach muscles and bring your right knee into your chest. Then slowly lower the foot back to the floor while keeping your low back in contact with the floor. Then tighten your stomach muscles and bring your left leg in. Go back and forth slowly for 8 to 12 repetitions on both sides.

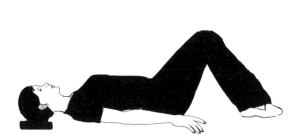 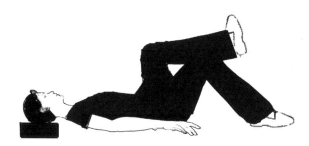

Checklist
✓   Make sure you keep your head and chin level
✓   Tighten your stomach every time your bring the knee in and as you lower the foot back down
✓   Keep your low back in contact with the floor throughout this exercise
✓   Use diaphragmatic breathing through the nose as much as possible
✓   Do not exercise to the point of strain or discomfort

Bridge

This exercise targets the abdominals and low back. Lie on the floor on your back with the knees bent, feet on the floor. Make sure you keep the head and neck level do not arch the head or tip the chin back. If you find that you are arching your neck, place a pillow under the head. Tighten the buttocks muscles and lift the hips off the floor as high as you can. Make sure you do not let the head tip back as you lift, keep the neck straight and the chin level. Keep both knees pointing straight up to the ceiling do not let the knees roll in or out.

Exhale as you lift the hips and inhale as you lower the hips. Repeat eight to twelve times. After completing eight to twelve repetitions hold for a stretch in the lifted position for five to ten deep belly breaths, or for as long as is comfortable.

Bridge Pose Down   Bridge Pose Up

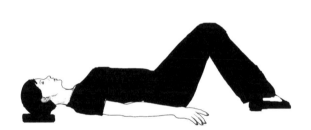
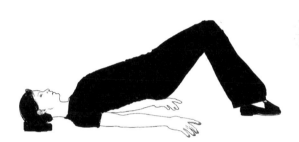

Checklist
✓ Make sure you keep your head and chin level
✓ Make sure you do not tip the head back when you lift the hips
✓ Keep the knees pointing up to the ceiling
✓ Use diaphragmatic breathing through the nose as much as possible
✓ Do not exercise to the point of strain or discomfort

Supine Leg Lift

Lie on the floor on your back with the knees bent, feet on the floor. Make sure you keep the head and neck level do not arch the head or tip the chin back. If you find that you are arching your neck, place a pillow under the head. Begin with a pelvic tilt.

Throughout this exercise make sure your low back stays in contact with the floor. Do not let the low back arch. Keeping the low back tight against the floor lift your right leg straight up. Tighten your abdominal muscles and slowly, with control lower your leg as close as you can to the floor keeping your low back pressed into the floor. Then slowly lift the leg back up. If the back begins to arch make the movement smaller. The further away from the floor that your leg is the easier it is to keep your back flat.

Make sure you keep the left knee bent and the left foot on the floor. Stretching your left leg out along the floor can cause back strain. You will find that as your abdominal muscles strengthen you will be able to lower your leg closer to the floor. Do eight to twelve repetitions and repeat with the left leg.

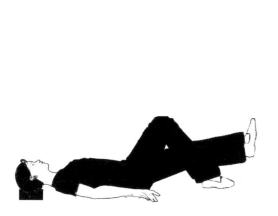 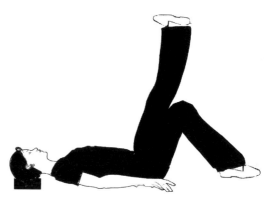

Checklist
➤ Make sure you keep your head and chin level
➤ Make sure you keep the low back in contact with the floor
➤ Keep the leg that is not moving bent with the foot on the floor. To prevent back injury avoid straightening both legs at the same time
➤ Use diaphragmatic breathing through the nose as much as possible
➤ Do not exercise to the point of strain or discomfort

Summary

There are many other exercises that work the same muscle groups, and many variations on the above exercises. There are also strengthening exercises that can be done using theraband, tubing, and physioballs, and your own body weight. The exercises listed in this chapter demonstrate a safe and complete workout and provide a good starting point. However, following the same exercise routine for long periods will eventually cause your body to adapt to the exercises, and you will discontinue getting good results. It is important to vary your exercise routine from time to time, trying different exercises and different forms of resistance.

After you become familiar with the various muscles you are trying to isolate and you become comfortable using resistance, try looking into other books, videos or classes to help vary your routine. When following any exercise program, remember to use good body mechanics and good form in order to protect your back and joints from injury.

Remember, resistance exercises should always be done slowly and with control.

Chapter Four

Yoga For Flexibility and Balance

"Excellence can be attained if you
Care more than others think is wise,
Risk more than others think is safe,
Dream more than others think is practical, and
Expect more than others think is possible."
- Claude T. Bissell

Balance problems are common in those with MS and they can increase the risk of a fall.

➢ Having MS can cause feelings of unsteadiness, being off-balance or dizziness, all of which can make walking or standing in place difficult.
➢ MS can cause your body to sway when trying to stand still and hinders the ability to safely climb up and down stairs or step up and down off of stools.
➢ The changes in balance common with MS can lead to taking short, quick shuffling steps when walking which increases the likelihood of a fall even more.
➢ Falls need to be prevented because those with MS who do fall are at a high risk of injuries which can negatively impact quality of life.

Along with having MS, falls can occur due to medications such as sedatives, muscle relaxants and blood pressure drugs, which can cause dizziness, lightheadedness, or loss of balance. When two or more medications are used in combination, these side effects may be aggravated. Other causes include diminished vision, hearing, muscle strength, coordination and reflexes. Carrying items when walking or not keeping your mind on walking and where you are going also increases the chances of a fall.

Falls often occur at home and are common when getting in and out of a chair or shower, stepping backwards, and reaching out too far to grab onto something. Having a fear of falling tends to lead to a restriction of movement and activities, which in turn makes you tighter and weaker, beginning a downward spiral. Instead of becoming less active, the goal is to focus on doing exercises that improve balance, strength and help to maintain function, thereby reducing the risk of falling.

Good balance is important to help you get around, remain independent, and carry out daily activities. Having good balance means being able to control and maintain your body's position whether you are moving or remaining still. An intact sense of balance helps you walk without staggering, rise from a chair without falling, and climb stairs more easily.

Exploring Balance

The body maintains balance by coordinating information received from three systems – vestibular, visual, and proprioceptive. The vestibular system works with the visual system to keep objects in focus when the head is moving. Joint and muscle receptors send signals to the brain to aid in maintaining balance. The brain receives, interprets, and processes the information from all of these systems in order to control balance.

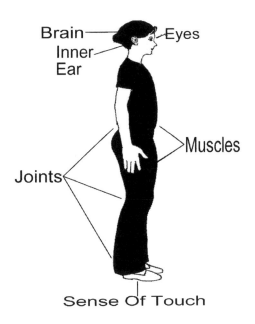

> ### *The vestibular or auditory system*

This system helps maintain balance by sensing the movement and position of the head, and acceleration and deceleration of the body. This occurs through the semicircular canals which are three tiny, fluid-filled tubes in your inner ear. Movement of fluid in the semicircular canals signals the brain about the direction, speed, and rotation of the head, such as when nodding up and down or looking from right to left. When the head moves, the liquid inside the semicircular canals also moves. This in turn puts pressure on the tiny hairs that line each canal. These hairs translate the movement of the liquid into nerve messages that are sent to your brain. Your brain then can tell your body how to stay balanced.

> *The visual system*

This system sends visual signals to the brain about the body's position in relation to its surroundings. These signals are processed by the brain and compared to information from the vestibular and the proprioceptive systems. The visual system provides the central nervous system with visual cues which are utilized as reference points in orienting the body in space.

> *The proprioceptive system*

This system provides an information link between your brain and the more than 650 muscles that move your body. This system relies on feedback from skin pressure and muscle and joint sensory receptors to tell the brain what part of the body is touching the ground and what parts of the body are moving. This system is made up of receptor cells found within each muscle fiber and nerves that travel from the muscles through the spinal cord to the brain. This system utilizes specific communication patterns within the brain that interpret these signals, allowing your body to meet the ever-changing demands of movement and balance. When this system is functioning efficiently an individual's body position is automatically adjusted in different situations. The proprioceptive system is responsible for providing the body with the necessary signals to allow us to plan and execute different motor tasks such as sitting properly in a chair and stepping off a curb smoothly. It also allows the body to coordinate fine motor movements such as writing with a pencil, using a spoon to drink soup, and buttoning one's shirt. In order for this system to work properly, it must rely on obtaining accurate information from the sensory systems and then organizing and interpreting this information efficiently and effectively.

Acting together, these three systems constantly gather and interpret information from all over the body and then act on that information in an appropriate and helpful way. The information from these systems travels to the central balance mechanism in your brain. In turn, the brain sends out signals allowing you to control your body movements, maintain your balance, and give you a sense of stability.

How Exercise Can Help

MS related falls are caused in part by a reduced sense of balance, a loss of ability to judge body placement and a loss of sensitivity in the proprioceptors. Slower reflexes, fatigue and decreased muscle strength also contribute to a diminished sense of equilibrium.

These changes in balance can be worsened due to a sedentary lifestyle. Failure to exercise regularly results in poor muscle tone, decreased strength and loss of bone mass and flexibility. All of the above can contribute to a fall and can have an impact on the severity of any injury that might occur as a result of a fall.

Maintaining balance requires stability of the core muscles and the joints, particularly the hip, knee, and ankle. With inactivity these areas can lose muscle strength and size.

Performing balance exercises challenges the proprioceptor system. As with any system in the body, when it is challenged it can improve. A mounting body of evidence indicates that balance training can improve one's strength, coordination, and muscle-reaction times.

The aerobic exercises in chapter two help to improve balance, as they challenge the body to move in a variety of directions at a quick pace, which can improve your reflexes. The strength training exercises in chapter three help to improve muscular strength that will provide more stability. The yoga movements in this chapter introduce static postures which will improve the body's ability to maintain balance while in various positions. While you may initially find these exercises challenging, with constant practice you will find your balance improving, thereby reducing your risk of a fall.

Exploring Flexibility and Range of Motion

Flexibility refers to the ability to move the joints and muscles through their full range of motion. Daily stretching can help to combat the muscular changes that accompanies MS. As you become more flexible and gain greater range of motion, you will find it easier to perform everyday activities such as reaching items on high shelves, looking behind you to back up the car, or tying your shoes.

Benefits of regular stretching include:
✓ Increased range of motion of joints.
✓ Better posture.
✓ Protection against muscle injuries such as strains or sprains.
✓ Improved circulation.
✓ Reduction in muscle tension.

Do's and Don'ts of Stretching
➢ Stretch only to the point where you feel a gentle pull.
➢ Do not stretch to the point of pain.
➢ *Do not bounce while you stretch.* Bouncing can cause small tears in muscle fibers that can lead to less flexibility.
➢ Do not hold your breath while you stretch. Breathe evenly in-and-out during each stretch.
➢ Hold each stretch approximately 30-45 seconds.

One benefit of stretching is that it increases the length of both your muscles and tendons, leading to an increase in range of movement. A flexible joint has the ability to move through a greater range of motion while requiring less energy to do so. Daily stretching improves muscular balance and posture. Stretching also increases joint synovial fluid, which is a lubricating fluid that promotes the transport of more nutrients to the joints' articular cartilage. This allows a greater range of motion and can reduce joint degeneration. Improved muscle coordination is another benefit of regular stretching. Research suggests that nerve-impulse velocity (the time it takes an impulse to travel to the brain and back) is improved with stretching.

Yoga

The practice of yoga is often misunderstood by many. The thought of yoga often conjures up thoughts of having to sit cross legged on the floor for long periods, standing on one's head, chanting, being connected with a particular religion or spiritual belief, or wrapping oneself into a posture which seems impossible for the average human to do.

Yoga is not about achieving advanced postures, sitting still for long periods, or being connected to a specific religious practice. The word yoga, taken from the Sanskrit word "*Yuj,*" simply means union; union of mind, body and spirit or soul, nothing more. The goal of yoga is to become more connected with your body and mind through the use of movement, breathwork and meditation or directed concentration.

The practice of yoga can help improve posture, balance, increase flexibility, reduce stress, lower blood pressure and aids in lessening common aches and pains. Yoga can be especially beneficial for those with injuries or chronic illness. Since yoga is about union of mind, body, and spirit, the main goal for the yoga student is to find the expression of the posture that best suits his or her individual and unique needs. It is about both a willingness to go inside to discover the movements that are best, and a willingness to honor those discoveries. Many traditional yoga postures can be adapted to accommodate all ability levels and ages. There are chair yoga classes in which every movement is performed sitting in a chair, and there are also programs for those who are bedridden. Yoga does not require one to follow any specific belief system to participate. The philosophies of yoga are universal and can be incorporated within any belief system.

Yoga can be a wonderful form of exercise, due to its slow and gentle nature. Many of the postures help improve balance and reduce the risk of falls. As the student of yoga gently and with respect for the body begins to increase flexibility, aches and pains in the back, knees, and hips may lessen as the muscles are stretched and the pressure exerted on the joints is reduced. Also, as flexibility increases, many of the activities of daily life become easier. When the muscles of the neck loosen it becomes easier to turn the head when trying to back up the car. When the muscles of the legs and back become more limber it becomes easier to reach or pick up items at varying heights. With an increased range of motion in the shoulder muscles, grooming and dressing tasks can become easier.

Below are some benefits of a yoga practice.

➢ Increased feelings of relaxation. Gentle stretching, breathing, meditation and guided relaxation releases body tension and calms the nervous system and emotions.

- ➢ Improved concentration. Focus, attention, and concentration are promoted through a yoga practice of mindful movement and enhanced body awareness.
- ➢ Muscle toning. Holding yoga postures is a form of isometric exercise that tones the muscles of the body.
- ➢ Improved flexibility. Yoga postures gently stretch the muscles in the body increasing the flexibility and length of the muscles, tendons and ligaments.
- ➢ Improved energy levels. Slow, gentle movements with deep breathing energize the body.
- ➢ Improved lung capacity. The deep diaphragmatic breathing encouraged in yoga can help to strengthen the lungs and improve respiratory health.

As with many of the movements in this book, the yoga postures will be shown standing, standing while holding on, and seated. Try to do as many postures as you can standing without holding on to begin to improve your balance.

Yoga and MS

One reason yoga is beneficial for those with MS is it's focus on deep diaphragmatic breathing. This is especially important if you are unable to achieve deep breathing through more vigorous aerobic exercise. Yoga based deep breathing can help to increase lung capacity, aid circulation, improve feelings of fatigue, and aid in maintaining respiratory health thereby diminishing the possibility of developing lung infections such as pneumonia.

You may need to adapt some or all of the postures to fit your needs. Props such as chairs, yoga straps, or towels can be helpful. Using a chair or wall for support for balance can also be helpful. You may find that with time and regular practice you will not need the props as much. All of the postures in this chapter are shown with some modifications – however you may need to find your own method to suit your individual needs. Remember, yoga is about discovering your body's unique needs and then adjusting your practice to honor those needs. If something does not feel right – do not do it. Do not ignore signals from your body that it is time to stop or go easier. With continued practice you may find the postures easier to do and feel positive changes in your body.

An important component of yoga is the combination of deep breathing and movement. The breath we will use with all of the postures is the same breath used throughout this book.

Belly Breathing Seated

Sit up straight and away from the back of the chair if possible.
Rest your hands across your abdomen.
As you exhale through the nose, gently contract your abdominal muscles and push all of the air out of your belly and lungs.

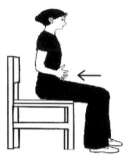

As you inhale through the nose let the belly rise first. Your belly and hands should move out with the inhalation. Then let the chest rise next. It may take some practice to have the belly move first. Do not let the shoulders rise up when inhaling. The shoulders stay down and relaxed the entire time.

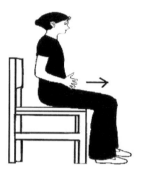

Yoga Poses

For all of the following postures *remember,* that yoga is about honoring the body's needs. With each posture experiment to find a level of intensity where you are challenging yourself but not struggling. If the breathing becomes restricted or the only thought you have is how soon you can release the posture, you are pushing yourself too hard. If you find the above happening, lessen the stretch or come out of the posture sooner.

The following movements should be done slowly and gently. Without forcing, try to increase your range of motion with each exhale. Do not push your body to do more than feels right. Since each day with MS can be different, each yoga session will be as well. Use this segment as an opportunity to notice which areas of your body are tight or uncomfortable, and which areas move more easily. This process will help you to determine which postures are appropriate to do, and how vigorous or gently you should proceed.

Half Neck Rolls

If possible sit at the front edge of the chair allowing your abdominal muscles to hold you up straight. If you are experiencing discomfort or find yourself slouching, slide all the way back in the chair so your back remains straight.

Drop your right ear to your right shoulder.

Circle your chin to your chest.

Circle your left ear to your left shoulder.

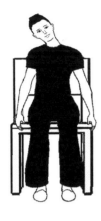 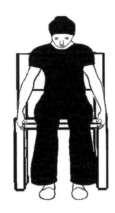 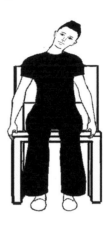

Reverse the movement making a half circle from left to right. It is not recommended to drop the head backwards as this compresses the neck.

Exhale as you circle your chin to your chest and inhale as you roll the ear to the shoulder. Use deep belly breathing through just the nose as much as possible.

Do this movement *slowly and gently*, counting *one-one thousand, two-one thousand, three-one thousand, four-one thousand* each time you circle your chin to your chest, and use the same count each time you roll the ear to the shoulder.

Do this movement 8-12 times. One repetition involves going to both sides.

Checklist
- ✓ Sit up straight
- ✓ Do not turn the head, look straight forward
- ✓ Move slowly using a 4 thousand count for each movement
- ✓ Exhale as you circle the chin to the chest, and inhale as you roll the ear to the shoulder
- ✓ Use diaphragmatic breathing through the nose as much as possible
- ✓ Do not exercise to the point of strain or discomfort

Neck Stretch

After circling 8-12 times, hold to the right, dropping the right ear to the right shoulder. Do not turn your head or chin, look straight forward to stretch the side of the neck. Each time you exhale let the right ear drop closer to the right shoulder and gently press the left shoulder down a bit more. Hold for 5-10 deep belly breaths.

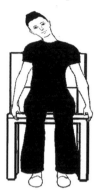

Next, hold to the left side, dropping the left ear to the left shoulder. Do not turn your head or chin, look straight forward to stretch the side of the neck. Each time you exhale let the left ear drop closer to the left shoulder and gently press the right shoulder down a bit more. Hold for 5-10 deep belly breaths.

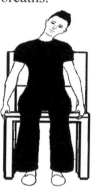

Next, drop the chin to the chest, and hold. Sit up straight. With each exhale roll the shoulders back and down and gently drop the chin, stretching the back of the neck. Hold for 5-10 deep belly breaths.

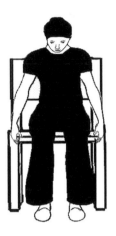

Checklist
✓ Sit up straight
✓ Do not turn the head, look straight forward
✓ Do this stretch once in each direction
✓ Hold each stretch for 5-10 deep belly breaths
✓ Use diaphragmatic breathing through the nose as much as possible
✓ Do not exercise to the point of strain or discomfort

Head Rotation

Bring the head back to a neutral position. Check to see that you are still sitting up straight and away from the back of the chair if possible.

Keeping your chin parallel to the floor, turn your head to the right to look over the right shoulder. Come back to center. Then turn the head to the left and look over the left shoulder. Come back to center.

Exhale each time you turn the head to the side. Inhale each time you come back to center.

Do this movement *slowly and gently*, counting *one-one thousand, two-one thousand, three-one thousand, four-one thousand* each time you turn to the side. Use the same count as you come back to the center, and again each time you turn the head to the other side.

Do this movement 8-12 times. One repetition involves going to both sides.

Turning the head to the right.   Turning the head to the left.

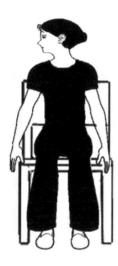   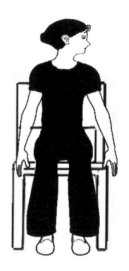

Checklist
- ✓ Sit up straight
- ✓ Move slowly using a 4 thousand count for each movement
- ✓ Use diaphragmatic breathing through the nose as much as possible
- ✓ Do not exercise to the point of strain or discomfort

Head Rotation Stretch

After completing 8-12 repetitions. Hold to the right side looking over the right shoulder. Each time you exhale see if you can look a bit more to the right and gently press the left shoulder back a bit more. Hold for 5-10 deep belly breaths.

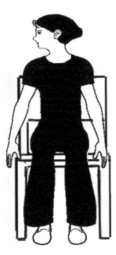

Then hold to the left side. Each time you exhale see if you can look a bit more to the left and gently press the right shoulder back a bit more. Hold for 5-10 deep belly breaths.

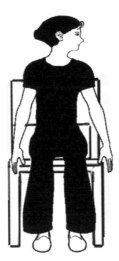

Checklist
- ✓ Sit up straight
- ✓ Do the stretches once in each direction
- ✓ Hold each stretch for 5-10 deep belly breaths
- ✓ Use diaphragmatic breathing through the nose as much as possible
- ✓ Do not exercise to the point of strain or discomfort

Shoulder Rolls

Bring the head back to a neutral position. Check to see if you are still sitting up straight and away from the back of the chair if possible.

Lift the shoulders up towards the ears as high as you can in a shrugging motion. Then roll the shoulders down and back, pressing them down as far as you can. Do this movement *slowly and gently,* counting *one-one thousand, two-one thousand, three-one thousand, four-one thousand* each time you lift the shoulders. Use the same count as you lower the shoulders.

Inhale as you lift the shoulders up and exhale as you press the shoulders down.

Exaggerate at both ends of the movement. Make sure you do not bend the elbows. The arms stay straight and the movement is all in the shoulders. This is an area which can become stiff, so it is helpful to have someone watch you do this movement to make sure the shoulders are both lifting up and pressing down.

Repeat for 8-12 shoulder rolls.

Press the shoulders down

Roll the shoulders up

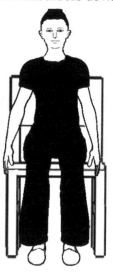 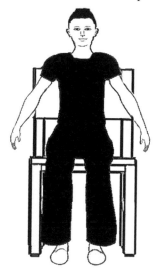

Checklist
- ✓ Sit up straight
- ✓ Use diaphragmatic breathing through the nose as much as possible
- ✓ Move slowly using a 4 thousand count for each movement
- ✓ Make sure you are lifting the shoulders up and lowering them down
- ✓ Do not bend the elbows, keep the arms straight
- ✓ Do not exercise to the point of strain or discomfort

Seated Spinal Twist

This movement will help to loosen the trunk muscles. If you have any sensitivities or injuries in your back such as osteoporosis or fractures you may wish to check with your health care provider about the appropriateness of twisting movements. Feeling a stretch or pull in the muscles can mean that you are stretching them, but you should never experience sharp or stabbing pain either during or after your exercise session. It is recommended that you do this movement very slowly with control and be aware of how it affects you. Remember, *never* go to the point of pain.

Sit up straight and away from the back of the chair if possible. Hold onto your elbows, keep the shoulders down away from the ears, and sit up straight. Begin to turn to the right, *turning at your waist.* Bring your arms and head with you. Turn to look over your right shoulder as far as you can. Come back to center and repeat to the left.

Do this movement *slowly and gently,* counting *one-one thousand, two-one thousand, three-one thousand, four-one thousand* each time you turn to the side. Use the same count as you turn back to the center. Inhale as you come to the center, and exhale as you turn to the side.

Do this movement 8 to 12. One repetition involves going to both sides.

Gently turn to the right Look over your right shoulder.	Center	Gently turn to the left Look over your left shoulder.
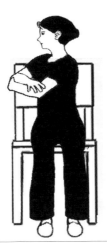	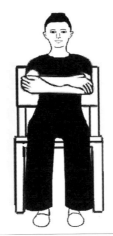	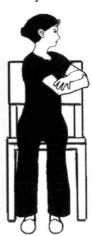

Checklist

➢ Sit up straight
➢ Use caution with twisting movements if you have back injuries or sensitivities
➢ Move slowly using a four thousand count for each movement
➢ Make sure you turn from the waist, not just the shoulders
➢ Turn your head to look back over your shoulder to complete the movement
➢ Use diaphragmatic breathing through the nose as much as possible
➢ Keep the shoulders down and back
➢ Do not exercise to the point of strain or discomfort

Seated Spinal Stretch

Check your posture before you begin. Shoulders should be back and down and over the hips. Tuck in the chin and think about pushing the crown of the head up to the ceiling without lifting your chin. The abdominal muscles are lightly pulled in, but not so much that it restricts your breathing.

Use caution with this posture if you have any sensitivities in the back. Check with your health care provider if you have concerns about the appropriateness of twisting movements.

Sit up straight away from the back of the chair if possible. Reach the left hand to the outside of the right knee. Turn to the right beginning the movement at the waist. Reach your right arm back behind you and look over your right shoulder. Turn as far as you comfortably can and look behind you as far as you can. You can press *gently* against your knee to help you twist further. Each time you inhale sit up straighter. Each time you exhale turn from the waist a little bit more. Hold for five to ten deep belly breaths, or for as long as is comfortable. Repeat with the right hand on the outside of the left knee.

Spinal Twist Right   Spinal Twist Left

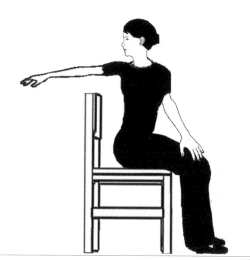
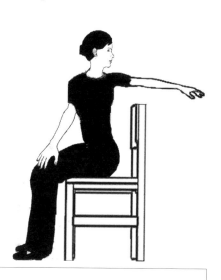

Checklist

- ➤ Sit up straight
- ➤ Use caution with twisting movements if you have back injuries or sensitivities
- ➤ Hold to each side for 5 to 10 breaths
- ➤ Make sure you turn from the waist, not just the shoulders
- ➤ Turn your head to look back over your shoulder to complete the movement
- ➤ Use diaphragmatic breathing through the nose as much as possible
- ➤ Keep the shoulders down and back
- ➤ Do not exercise to the point of strain or discomfort

Chest Opener

This movement is helpful to stretch the shoulders and open the chest. If you have any sensitivities in your shoulders do this movement gently until you know how it will affect your shoulders.

Check that you are sitting up straight and away from the back of the chair if possible. Clasp your hands behind your head or neck. Do not pull the head forward, keep your neck in alignment. If you can not bring your hands together behind your neck, you can bring your fingertips to the sides of your head. As you continue these stretches, you may find that your flexibility increases.

Bring the elbows to the front as close together as you can. Again, do not pull the head forward; just go as far as you can with good alignment.

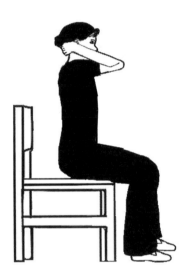

Next, open the shoulders up, bringing the elbows back as far as you comfortably can. Let the chest come forward and the low back arch slightly. Gently press the back of the head into the hands and squeeze the shoulder blades together in the back. Keep the shoulders down away from the ears.

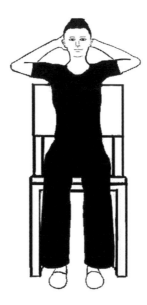

Inhale as you open the elbows, and exhale as the elbows come together.

Do this movement *slowly and gently, counting one-one thousand, two-one thousand, three-one thousand, four-one thousand* each time you open the elbows, and use the same count each time you bring the elbows together.

Do this movement 8-12 times.

Try to take deep breaths as you bring the elbows back. This movement opens the chest allowing the lungs to fully expand.

Checklist
✓ Sit up straight
✓ Move slowly using a 4 thousand count for each movement
✓ Use diaphragmatic breathing through the nose as much as possible
✓ Do not pull your head forward with your hands
✓ Do not exercise to the point of strain or discomfort

Chest Stretch

This movement will help to open the chest and the shoulders and it is helpful for correcting posture. This stretch is good after working at a desk or computer for some time. Check your posture before you begin. Shoulders should be back and down and over the hips. Tuck the chin in and think about pushing the crown of the head up to the ceiling without lifting your chin. The abdominal muscles are lightly pulled in, but not so much as to restrict your breathing.

If you can, clasp your hands behind your back. If you are unable to clasp your hands, just reach back. Draw your shoulder blades together and lift your hands away from your body as far as you can without hurting your shoulders. Be careful to not lean forward as you lift your hands. Your shoulders should stay over your hips. Hold for 5-10 deep belly breaths or to comfort.

Standing   Seated

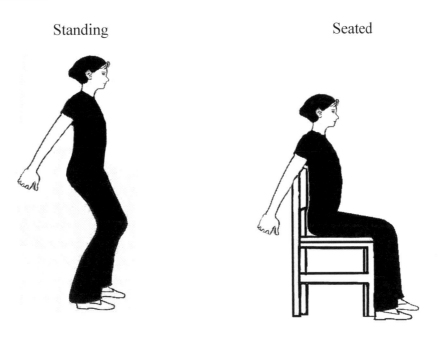

Checklist
✔ Stand or sit up straight
✔ Use diaphragmatic breathing through the nose as much as possible
✔ Keep the knees slightly bent when standing
✔ Do not lean forward as you lift the arms
✔ Do not exercise to the point of strain or discomfort

Arm Circles

This movement will help to loosen the shoulders. Check your posture before you begin. Shoulders should be back and down and over the hips. Knees should remain slightly bent. Tuck the chin in and think about pushing the crown of the head up to the ceiling without lifting your chin. The abdominal muscles are lightly pulled in, but not so much as to restrict your breathing.

Lift both arms out to the side, shoulder height if you can. Turn the palms so they face up to the ceiling. Push the hands out to both sides to lengthen the arms and try to straighten the elbows without locking them. Move the hands back as far as you can to open the chest, but not so far as to cause discomfort in your shoulders. Holding here, make five small arm circles *backwards*. Focus on going backwards in order to open the chest and shoulders. Circling forwards can cause rounding of the shoulders, the exact postural habit that we are trying to change. Then relax your arms down by your sides. Repeat three to five more times.

Standing   Seated

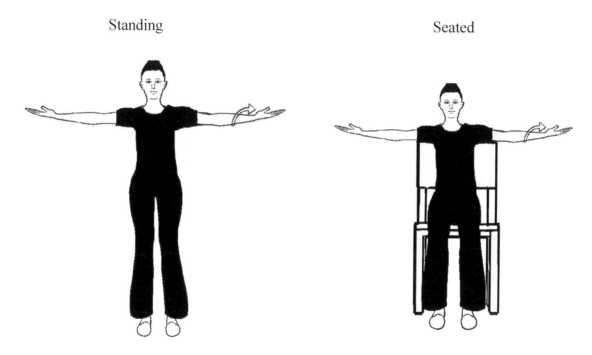

Checklist
- Stand or sit up straight
- Use diaphragmatic breathing through the nose as much as possible
- Keep the knees slightly bent
- Make sure you circle the arms backwards, not forwards
- Stretch your arms out to the sides and bring them back as far as you can to open the chest
- Do not exercise to the point of strain or discomfort

Overhead Stretch

This movement helps to loosen the shoulders and open the chest. Check your posture before you begin. Shoulders should be back and down and over the hips. Knees should remain slightly bent. Tuck the chin in and think about pushing the crown of the head up to the ceiling without lifting your chin. The abdominal muscles are lightly pulled in, but not so much as to restrict your breathing.

Lift your arms up overhead clasping the fingers if possible. If you can not go that far just reach your arms up. Turn your hands so your palms face the ceiling. Press your palms up to the ceiling, try to straighten your elbows, but do not lock them. Bring the arms back towards your ears as far as you can, without hurting your shoulders. Hold for five to ten deep belly breaths. Each time you inhale try to stretch up further, draw the arms back and straighten the elbows. Each time you exhale relax the shoulders. Repeat five more times.

Standing   Seated

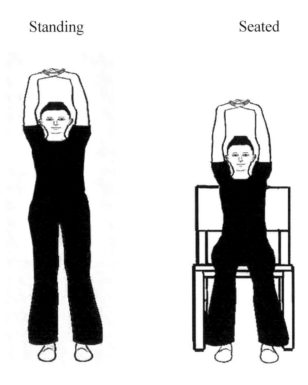

Checklist
➤ Stand or sit up straight
➤ Use diaphragmatic breathing through the nose as much as possible
➤ Keep the knees slightly bent when standing
➤ Do not exercise to the point of strain or discomfort

The next few movements are helpful if you have been sitting for some time. Many falls happen while transitioning from sitting to standing. Sitting for long periods can reduce the circulation in the legs, impairing balance. These ankle exercises will help restore circulation to the legs.

Toe Lifts

Check that you are sitting up straight and away from the back of the chair if possible. Keeping the heels on the floor, lift both toes off the floor as high as you can. Repeat 8-12 times.

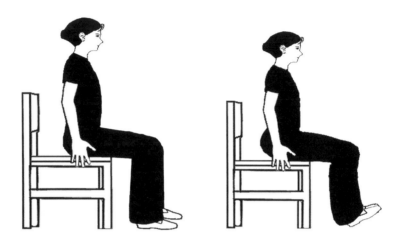

Heel Lifts

Check that you are sitting up straight and away from the back of the chair if possible. Keeping the toes on the floor, lift both heels off the floor as high as you can. Repeat 8-12 times.

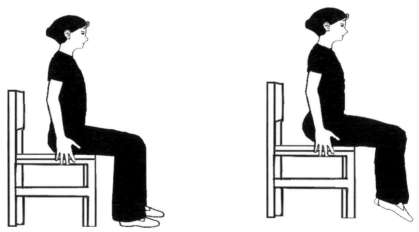

You can also alternate between these two movements i.e., lift the toes and then the heels, and continue back and forth.

Ankle Circles

Check your posture before you begin. Shoulders should be back and down and over the hips. Tuck in the chin and think about pushing the crown of the head up to the ceiling without lifting your chin. The abdominal muscles are lightly pulled in, but not so much that it restricts your breathing.

Sit up straight and away from the back of the chair if possible. Lift the right foot slightly off the floor. Circle the ankle in one direction, and then the other. Be careful to circle just the ankle and not the whole leg. Repeat 8-12 times each way, taking deep belly breaths. Repeat with the left foot.

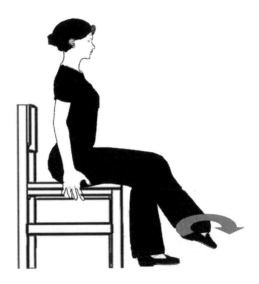

Checklist

✓ Sit up straight
✓ Keep the shoulders down away from the ears
✓ Keep the natural curve in the low back
✓ Make sure you circle just the ankle and not the whole leg
✓ Use diaphragmatic breathing through the nose as much as possible
✓ Do not exercise to the point of strain or discomfort

Standing Postures

The next few exercises are illustrated in a standing position, standing and holding on or seated on a chair or ball. Do as much as you can standing, but if you choose to sit, keep checking that you are sitting up straight and with good posture.

Mountain Pose

Check your posture before you begin. Shoulders should be back and down and over the hips. Knees should remain slightly bent. Tuck in the chin and think about pushing the crown of the head up to the ceiling without lifting your chin. The abdominal muscles are lightly pulled in, but not so much that it restricts your breathing.

Stand up straight and lift your arms up overhead with the palms facing each other. Bring the arms back so the elbows are in line with the ears if possible. Drop the shoulders and line the shoulders up over the hips. Keep the knees slightly bent and the natural curve in the low back. Toes point straight forward. Place equal weight on both feet. Check that there is equal weight on the outside and inside of the foot, and on all of the toes so you are not rolling your ankles in or out. Check that there is equal weight on the ball and heel of the foot so you are not leaning forward or back. Hold for 5-10 deep belly breaths, or to comfort.

Standing   *Standing with assistance*   *Seated*

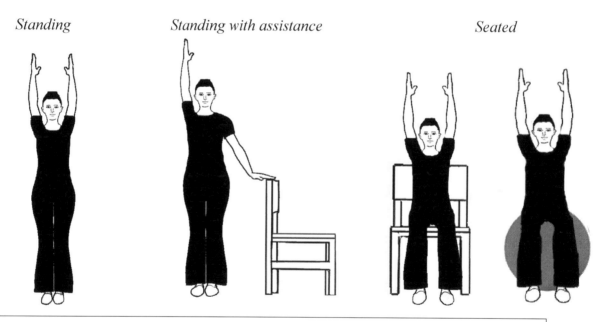

Checklist
✓ Stand or sit up straight, away from the back of the chair if possible
✓ Keep the spine straight and the shoulders over the hips
✓ Keep the shoulders down away from the ears
✓ Keep the knees slightly bent and the natural curve in the low back
✓ Hold for 5-10 deep belly breaths, or to comfort
✓ Use diaphragmatic breathing through the nose as much as possible
✓ Do not exercise to the point of strain or discomfort
✓ Remember the goal of yoga is to find that point where you are challenging yourself but not struggling

132

Warrior I Pose

Check your posture before you begin. Shoulders should be back and down and over the hips. Knees should remain slightly bent. Tuck in the chin and think about pushing the crown of the head up to the ceiling without lifting your chin. The abdominal muscles are lightly pulled in, but not so much that it restricts your breathing.

To start step your left leg back into a lunge position. Both feet should be pointing straight forward; do not turn your back foot or leg out to the side. Make sure that your right knee does not extend past your right ankle bone. You should be able to look down at your right knee and see both your right toes and the arch of the right foot. If you need a deeper stretch step the feet wider apart rather then lunging the right knee beyond the front toes. This will help to protect the knee joint from injury.

Lift the back heel off of the floor. Bring the hips under the shoulders, do not lean the upper body forward. Gently pull the right hip back, as you bring the left hip forward. Without lifting the shoulders, reach the arms out in front of you, with the palms facing each other. Hold for 5-10 deep belly breaths, or to comfort. Repeat on the left side.

Standing   *Standing with assistance*

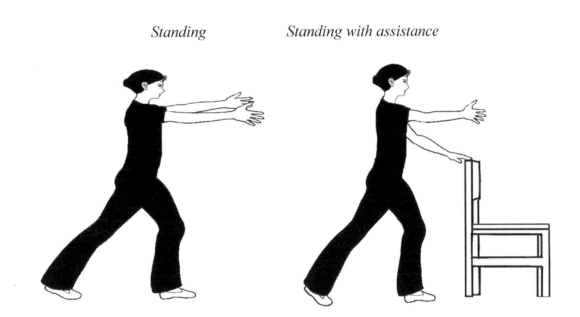

Seated

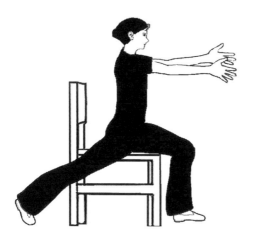 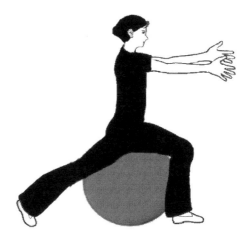

Checklist

✓ Stand or sit up straight
✓ Keep the spine straight and the shoulders over the hips
✓ Keep the shoulders down away from the ears
✓ Keep the knees slightly bent and the natural curve in the low back
✓ Keep the front knee aligned over the front ankle
✓ Hold for 5-10 deep belly breaths, or to comfort
✓ Use diaphragmatic breathing through the nose as much as possible
✓ Do not exercise to the point of strain or discomfort
✓ Remember the goal of yoga is to find that point where you are challenging yourself but not struggling

Warrior II Pose

Check your posture before you begin. Shoulders should be back and down and over the hips. Knees should remain slightly bent. Tuck in the chin and think about pushing the crown of the head up to the ceiling without lifting your chin. The abdominal muscles are lightly pulled in, but not so much that it restricts your breathing.

Step your right foot out to the side into a lunge position. The back knee is straight, but not locked and the front knee is bent. Turn the toes of the left foot in, so the left foot is at about a 45-degree angle. Turn the right toes out to the right side.

Make sure that your right knee does not extend past your right ankle bone. You should be able to look down at your right knee and see both your right toes and the arch of the right foot. Also check that your right knee is directly over your ankle and not rolling in or out. If you need a deeper stretch step the feet wider apart rather then lunging the right knee forward beyond the toes. This will help to protect the knee joint from injury.

Bring the arms out to the side about shoulder height with the palms facing the floor. Look out over your right hand. Bring the hips under the shoulders, do not lean the upper body forward. Hold for 5-10 deep belly breaths, or to comfort. Repeat on the left side.

Standing   *Standing with assistance*

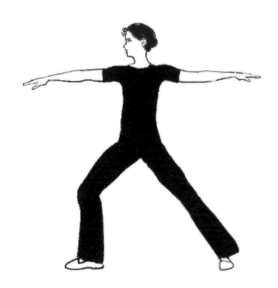 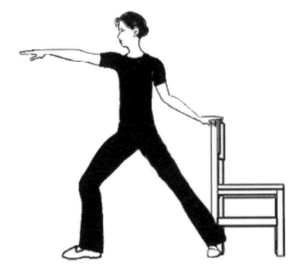

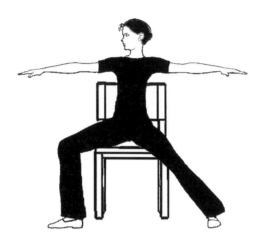
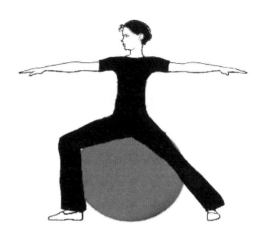

Checklist

✓ Stand or sit up straight
✓ Keep the spine straight and the shoulders over the hips
✓ Keep the shoulders down away from the ears
✓ Keep the knees slightly bent and the natural curve in the low back
✓ Keep the bent knee aligned over the ankle
✓ Hold for 5-10 deep belly breaths, or to comfort
✓ Use diaphragmatic breathing through the nose as much as possible
✓ Do not exercise to the point of strain or discomfort
✓ Remember the goal of yoga is to find that point where you are challenging yourself but not struggling

Lateral Angle Pose

Check your posture before you begin. Shoulders should be back and down and over the hips. Knees should remain slightly bent. Tuck in the chin and think about pushing the crown of the head up to the ceiling without lifting your chin. The abdominal muscles are lightly pulled in, but not so much that it restricts your breathing.

Step your right foot out to the side into a lunge position. The back knee is straight but not locked, and the front knee is bent. Turn the toes of the left foot in, so the foot is at about a 45-degree angle. Turn the right toes out to the right side.

Make sure that your right knee does not extend past your right ankle bone. You should be able to look down at your right knee and see both your right toes and the arch of the right foot. Also check that your right knee is directly over your ankle and not rolling in or out. If you need a deeper stretch step the feet wider apart rather then lunging the right knee forward beyond the toes.

Reach out to the right and bring your right hand (or for a deeper stretch your right elbow) to your right knee. Drop the left hip down making a straight line from your heel to your shoulder. Look up at your left hand if possible. If this is too strenuous just look straight ahead. Draw the left arm back to open the chest. *Do not lean the upper body forward.* Hold for 5-10 deep belly breaths, or to comfort. Repeat on the left side.

Standing   *Standing with assistance*

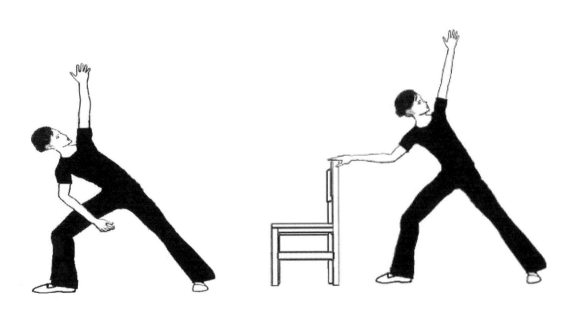

Placing the hand on the seat of the chair

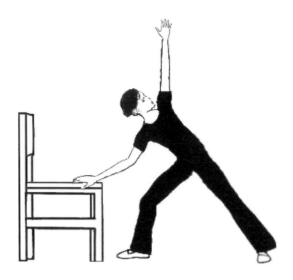

Seated

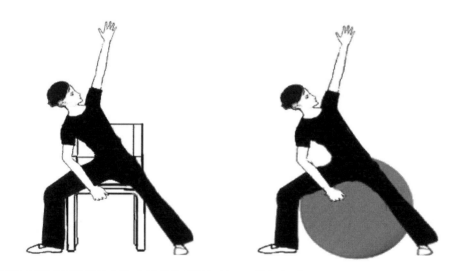

Checklist
- ✓ Stand or sit up straight
- ✓ Keep the shoulders down away from the ears
- ✓ Keep the knees slightly bent and the natural curve in the low back
- ✓ Keep the front knee aligned over the front ankle
- ✓ Hold for 5-10 deep belly breaths, or to comfort
- ✓ Use diaphragmatic breathing through the nose as much as possible
- ✓ Do not exercise to the point of strain or discomfort
- ✓ Remember the goal of yoga is to find that point where you are challenging yourself but not struggling

138

Warrior III Pose

The next few poses are balance poses and you should try to do them standing if possible. They are very difficult to do on a ball so seated versions are shown in a chair.

Check your posture before you begin. Shoulders should be back and down and over the hips. Knees should remain slightly bent. Tuck in the chin and think about pushing the crown of the head up to the ceiling without lifting your chin. The abdominal muscles are lightly pulled in, but not so much that it restricts your breathing.

Without raising the shoulders up, bring your arms up in front of you about shoulder height with the palms facing each other. Begin to lift the right leg up straight behind you.

The shoulders can tip *slightly* forward, but keep the body in a straight line from the heel to the head. Keep the natural curve in the low back. Lift the back leg as much as your balance allows.

Do not lift the leg so high that you cause discomfort in the low back. The purpose of this posture is to challenge your ability to stand on one foot, and should not cause back pain. The left knee (the leg you are standing on) should not be locked. Hold for 5-10 deep belly breaths, or to comfort. Repeat on the left.

Standing *Standing with assistance*

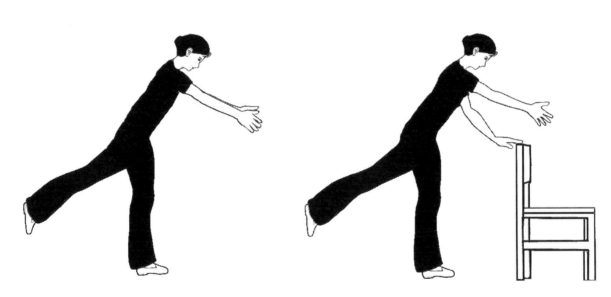

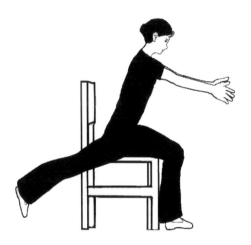

Checklist
- ✓ Stand or sit up straight
- ✓ Keep the shoulders down away from the ears
- ✓ Keep the knees slightly bent and the natural curve in the low back
- ✓ Do not lift the leg too high creating back pain
- ✓ Do not drop the shoulders too far forward
- ✓ Hold for 5-10 deep belly breaths, or to comfort
- ✓ Use diaphragmatic breathing through the nose as much as possible
- ✓ Do not exercise to the point of strain or discomfort
- ✓ Remember the goal of yoga is to find that point where you are challenging yourself but not struggling

Tree Pose

Check your posture before you begin. Shoulders should be back and down and over the hips. Knees should remain slightly bent. Tuck in the chin and think about pushing the crown of the head up to the ceiling without lifting your chin. The abdominal muscles are lightly pulled in, but not so much that it restricts your breathing.

Without raising the shoulders up, lift your arms up overhead with the palms facing each other. Shift your weight into the left leg. Place the sole of the right foot against the inside of the left leg. The higher you lift the right foot, the more challenging this posture is. Do not place the right foot directly on the side of the left knee in order to protect the joint.

You may wish to start by bringing the right foot to the left ankle bone while keeping the right toes on the floor. Bring the hips under the shoulders. Keep the natural curve in the low back. Lift the leg as high as your balance allows. The left knee (the leg you are standing on) should not be locked. Your right foot should be below or above the knee joint. Hold for 5-10 deep belly breaths, or to comfort. Repeat on the left.

Standing   *Standing with assistance*   *Seated*

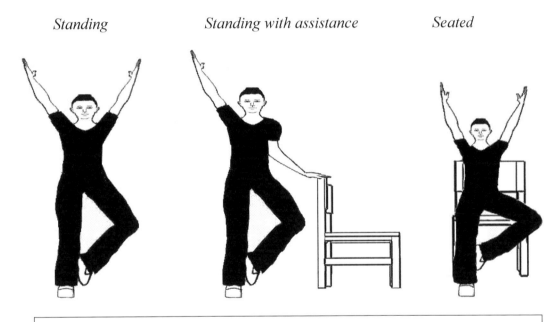

Checklist
✓ Stand or sit up straight
✓ Keep the shoulders down away from the ears
✓ Keep the hips under the shoulders
✓ Keep the knees slightly bent and the natural curve in the low back
✓ Hold for 5-10 deep belly breaths, or to comfort
✓ Use diaphragmatic breathing through the nose as much as possible
✓ Do not exercise to the point of strain or discomfort
✓ Remember the goal of yoga is to find that point where you are challenging yourself but not struggling

Dancer's Pose/Quadriceps Stretch

Check your posture before you begin. Shoulders should be back and down and over the hips. Tuck in the chin and think about pushing the crown of the head up to the ceiling without lifting your chin. The abdominal muscles are lightly pulled in, but not so much that it restricts your breathing.

Shift your weight into the left leg. Bend the right knee, bringing the heel as close to the buttocks as you can. Bring the hips under the shoulders. Bring the knees together and let the right knee point down towards the floor as much as possible.

If it is comfortable to do so, hold onto your right ankle, sock or pant leg. If this is creates too deep of a stretch just lift the heel back. Hold for five to ten deep belly breaths, or for as long as is comfortable. Repeat on the left.

Standing Holding Foot   Standing Modified

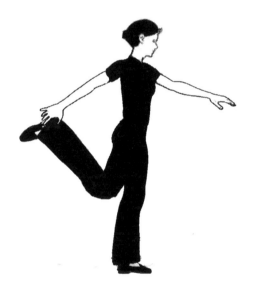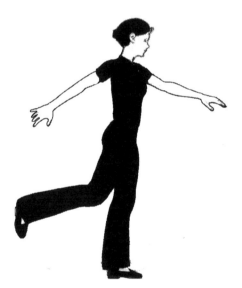

Standing with assistance

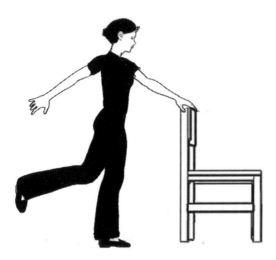

Seated

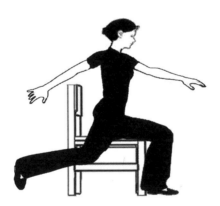

Checklist

- ✔ Stand or sit up straight
- ✔ Keep the shoulders down away from the ears
- ✔ Keep the hips under the shoulders
- ✔ Keep the knees slightly bent and the natural curve in the low back
- ✔ Hold for five to ten deep belly breaths, or to comfort
- ✔ Use diaphragmatic breathing through the nose as much as possible
- ✔ Remember the goal of yoga is to find that point where you are challenging yourself but not struggling

Floor Exercises

Floor exercises can be very beneficial for those with MS. The floor is a solid surface that provides feedback as to whether or not the back is straight. Doing floor exercises also keeps you in the habit of getting up and down. You may find that you will be able to get up more easily after a fall if you have been practicing getting up from the floor. Please refer to pages 32-33 for instructions as to how to get up and down safely.

Performing these exercises on a couch or bed is not as beneficial as these surfaces are often too soft. seated variations are also shown for days when you do not wish to get on the floor. If you choose to do floor exercises it is helpful to maintain a pelvic tilt in the back in order to protect the back from injury.

Knee To Chest Pose

Sit towards the front edge of the chair and lean your upper back against the chair. Keep the abdominal muscles contracted to help protect your back.

Draw your right knee up towards your chest and if possible hold underneath the knee. Be careful not to hold in front of the knee as this will compress the joint. If your hands will not reach under your right knee, you can wrap a towel or strap under the foot and hold the ends with your hands. Hold for five to ten deep belly breaths, or for as long as is comfortable. Repeat with the left knee.

Knee To Chest Sit   Knee To Chest Sit With Towel

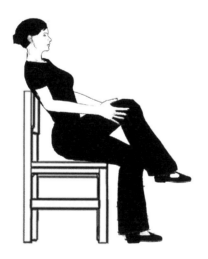
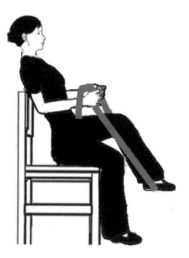

Floor variation

Lie on the floor on your back. Make sure you keep the head and neck level do not arch the head or tip the chin back. If you find that you are arching your neck, place a pillow under the head. Begin with a pelvic tilt (pg. 105). Throughout this exercise make sure your low back stays in contact with the floor.

Without arching the back bring your right knee towards your chest. You can either hold the knee with your hands or wrap a towel or yoga strap around the knee and hold the ends of the strap with your hands. When holding the knee make sure you hold under the knee and not on top of the knee so you do not compress the joint.

Make sure your head stays on the floor or pillow. Do not hold the head off the floor just to reach your knee as this strains the neck. *Do not pull the leg in hard, just bring the knee in enough until you feel a gentle stretch in the back of the leg you are holding up.* Hold for 5-10 deep belly breaths or to comfort. Repeat with the other leg.

Knee to Chest   Modification with Towel

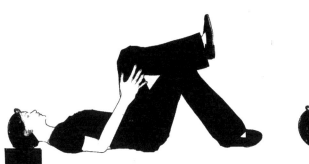 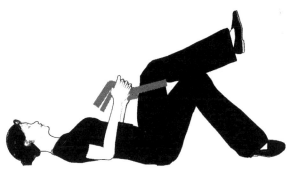

Checklist
- ✓ If seated, sit up straight and keep the shoulders down away from the ears
- ✓ If on the floor make sure you keep your head and chin level and your head on the floor or pillow
- ✓ Make sure you keep the low back in contact with the floor
- ✓ Make sure you hold underneath the knee not on top to avoid compressing the knee joint
- ✓ Use diaphragmatic breathing through the nose as much as possible
- ✓ Hold for 5-10 deep belly breaths, or to comfort
- ✓ Do not exercise to the point of strain or discomfort
- ✓ Remember the goal of yoga is to find that point where you are challenging yourself but not struggling

Hamstring Stretch/Seated Forward Bend Pose
Seated variation
Sit at the front edge of the chair. Extend your right leg forward and pull the toes towards you. Keep the back straight and bring your chest forward, hinging at the hips. Do not round your back as you come forward. Hold for five to ten deep belly breaths or for as long as is comfortable. Repeat with the other leg.

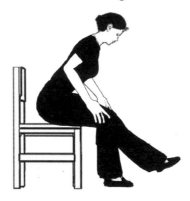

Floor Variation
Press your low back into the floor. Straighten your right leg and flex your foot but do not lock the knee. If this bothers your low back you can also leave a soft bend in the knee. You can either leave your hands by your sides on the floor or wrap a towel or yoga strap around the foot and hold the ends with your hands. Keep your head on the floor or pillow and do not hold the head off the floor just to hold the leg. Hold for five to ten deep belly breaths or for as long as is comfortable. Repeat with the other leg.

Hamstring Stretch Arms By Side   Hamstring Stretch Using a Towel

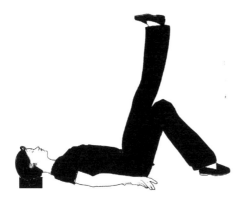 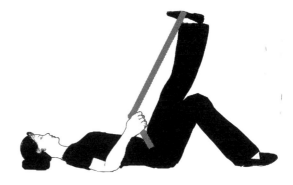

Checklist
- ✓ If seated, sit up straight and keep the ears away from the shoulders, keep the back straight as you lean forward, do not round the back
- ✓ Make sure you keep your head and chin level and your head on the floor or pillow
- ✓ Make sure you keep the low back in contact with the floor
- ✓ The knee can be straight or have a soft bend, do not lock the knee
- ✓ Use diaphragmatic breathing through the nose as much as possible
- ✓ Hold for 5-10 deep belly breaths
- ✓ Remember the goal of yoga is to find that point where you are challenging yourself but not struggling

Inner Thigh Stretch

Seated variation

Sit against the back of the chair. Wrap the strap around your right foot. Turn the leg out slightly and carry the leg out to the side until you feel a pull in your right inner thigh. Hold for five to ten deep belly breaths then repeat other leg.

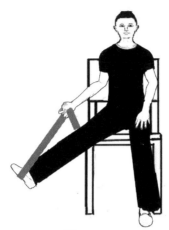

Floor variation

Wrap a towel or yoga strap around the right foot and hold the ends with your right hand. Let the leg drop out to the right. If it is comfortable to do so you can let the left hip roll off the floor and let the right foot rest on the floor. If this bothers your back, stay in a pelvic tilt and do not drop the foot to the floor. Hold for 5-10 deep belly breaths or to comfort. Repeat with the other leg.

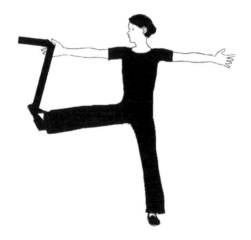

Checklist
- ✓ If seated, sit up straight and keep the ears away from the shoulders
- ✓ If on the floor, keep your head and chin level and your head on the floor or pillow
- ✓ The knee can be straight or have a soft bend, do not lock the knee
- ✓ Use diaphragmatic breathing through the nose as much as possible
- ✓ Hold for 5-10 deep belly breaths
- ✓ Remember the goal of yoga is to find that point where you are challenging yourself but not struggling

147

Outer Hip Stretch

Sit up straight against the back of the chair. Use caution with this exercise if you have had a hip replacement or have significant hip pain. If you have had a hip replacement, check with your healthcare provider about the appropriateness of this stretch. If in doubt follow the instructions for the modification.

Bring your right ankle bone up to the left knee. Let the right knee drop out to the side as much as possible. Make sure that you are not just crossing the legs. It should be your right ankle bone on your left knee, not your right knee. Hold for 5-10 deep belly breaths, or to comfort. Repeat with the left leg.

Modification: Cross your right ankle over your left ankle and let both knees fall out to the side as much as possible. Then repeat with the left ankle over the right.

Seated Hip Stretch   Modification

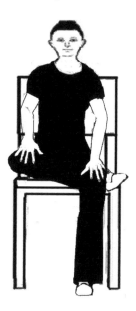
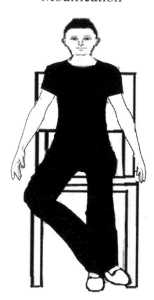

Floor variation

Press your low back into the floor wrap a towel or yoga strap around your right foot and hold the ends of the towel or strap with your left hand. Let the leg drop to the left, across the body. If it is comfortable to do so you can let the right hip roll off the floor and let the right foot rest on the floor. If this bothers your back, stay in a pelvic tilt and do not drop the foot to the floor. Hold for 5-10 deep belly breaths or to comfort. Repeat with the other leg.

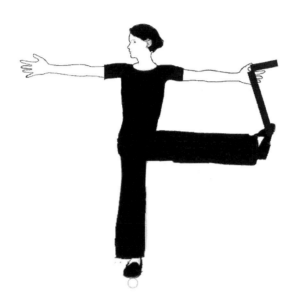

Checklist
- ✓ If seated, sit up straight and keep the shoulders down away from the ears
- ✓ If on the floor make sure you keep your head and chin level and your head on the floor or pillow
- ✓ If seated check that you are not just crossing the legs
- ✓ Hold for 5-10 deep belly breaths, or to comfort
- ✓ Use diaphragmatic breathing through the nose as much as possible
- ✓ Do not exercise to the point of strain or discomfort
- ✓ Remember the goal of yoga is to find that point where you are challenging yourself but not struggling

Spinal Twist

The next few postures are shown on the floor only as this allows you to completely relax into the stretch.

Lie on the floor on your back with the knees bent, feet on the floor. Make sure you keep the head and neck level do not arch the head or tip the chin back. If you find that you are arching your neck, place a pillow under the head.

Bring your arms out to the side in a "T" position with the palms facing the ceiling. Slowly lower both knees to the right. You can let your left hip roll off the floor and let the knees come to the floor. If that bothers your back stay in a pelvic tilt and do not drop the knees as far down.

Looking towards the knees is a gentler stretch, looking away from the knees is a deeper stretch.

Hold for 5-10 deep belly breaths. Repeat other side.

Spinal Twist Right   Spinal Twist Left

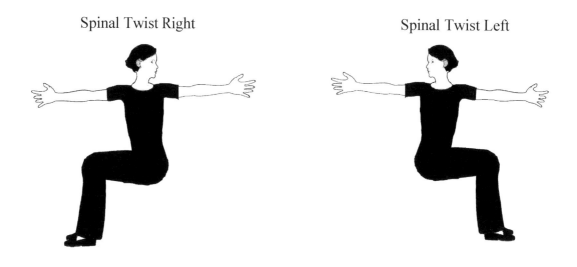

Checklist
- ✓ Only twist as far as it is comfortable to do so   use caution if your back is sensitive
- ✓ Use diaphragmatic breathing through the nose as much as possible
- ✓ Do not exercise to the point of strain or discomfort
- ✓ Remember the goal of yoga is to find that point where you are challenging yourself but not struggling

The next series of exercises are shown lying on the stomach. Many of us spend much of our day with the shoulders rounded forward as we go about daily tasks. This can cause the upper back muscles to become weak and over-stretched and the chest muscles to become tight. These postures are beneficial to help strengthen the upper back muscles and stretch the chest muscles to help correct posture.

Be gentle if your back is sensitive. You can modify these postures by placing a pillow under the hips which will lessen the arch in the low back. You may find that at first you need to use a pillow and then as the back strengthens you can do the postures without the pillow. Another modification is to place a rolled towel under the forehead if you find that lying with the face down is uncomfortable.

Prone Arm Lift

Lie on your stomach with the hands overhead, palms facing the floor, and feet relaxed. Place your forehead or chin on the floor. To protect the neck do not turn your head to the side. If needed, you can place a pillow under the hips (if your back is sensitive) or a towel roll under the forehead. Press your abdominal muscles and pelvic bones down into the floor and tighten the buttocks muscles. This will help to protect the back.

Lift just the right arm straight up off the floor. The elbow should be near your ear. Do not let the arm drift off to the side. Squeeze the shoulders blades together. Keep your other hand and both feet relaxed on the floor. Keep the head on the floor. The goal is to learn to work only one area of your body at a time while being able to relax the rest of your body. Try to avoid tightening the muscles of your left arm or lifting the legs off the floor. Hold for 5-10 deep belly breaths or to comfort. Relax and repeat with the left arm.

Lift just the right arm off the floor.
You can place a towel under the forehead or a pillow under the hips if needed.

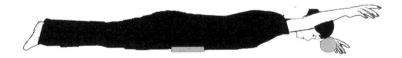

Checklist
✓ Press the stomach and hips into the floor and tighten the buttocks muscles to protect the back
✓ Lift just one arm at a time. Do not lift the other arm, feet, or head off the floor
✓ Use a pillow under the hips &/or towel roll under the forehead if needed
✓ Use diaphragmatic breathing through the nose as much as possible
✓ Do not exercise to the point of strain or discomfort
✓ Remember the goal of yoga is to find that point where you are challenging yourself but not struggling

Prone Leg Lift

Lie on your stomach with the hands overhead, palms facing the floor, and feet relaxed. Place your forehead or chin on the floor. To protect the neck do not turn your head to the side. If needed, you can place a pillow under the hips (if your back is sensitive) or a towel roll under the forehead. Press your abdominal muscles and pelvic bones down into the floor and tighten the buttocks muscles. This will help to protect the back.

Lift just the right leg straight up off the floor. Keep the knee as straight as you can. Keep your other leg and both arms relaxed on the floor. Keep the head on the floor. Squeeze the buttocks muscles as you lift. You should not feel a strain in your low back. Only lift the leg as high as you can without hurting your back. Try to avoid tightening the muscles of your left leg or lifting the arms off the floor.

Hold for 5-10 deep belly breaths or to comfort. Relax and repeat with the left leg.

Lift just the right leg off the floor.
You can place a towel under the forehead or a pillow under the hips if needed.

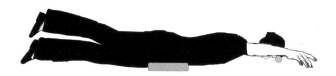

Checklist
- ✓ Press the stomach and hips into the floor and tighten the buttocks muscles to protect the back
- ✓ Lift just one leg at a time. Do not lift the other leg, arms, or head off the floor
- ✓ Use a pillow under the hips &/or towel roll under the forehead if needed
- ✓ Do not lift the leg too high and strain the low back
- ✓ Use diaphragmatic breathing through the nose as much as possible
- ✓ Do not exercise to the point of strain or discomfort
- ✓ Remember the goal of yoga is to find that point where you are challenging yourself but not struggling

Half Boat Pose

Lie on your stomach with the hands overhead, palms facing the floor, and feet relaxed. Place your forehead or chin on the floor. To protect the neck do not turn your head to the side. If needed, you can place a pillow under the hips (if your back is sensitive) or a towel roll under the forehead. Press your abdominal muscles and pelvic bones down into the floor and tighten the buttocks muscles. This will help to protect the back.

Lift just the right arm and left leg straight up off the floor. The right elbow should be near your ear. Do not let the arm drift off to the side. Keep the knee as straight as you can. Keep your left arm and right leg relaxed on the floor. Keep the head on the floor. Squeeze the shoulders blades together and tighten the buttocks muscles. You should not feel strain in your low back. Only lift the arm and leg as high as you can without hurting your back.

Try to avoid tightening the muscles of your left arm or right leg or lifting them off the floor. Hold for 5-10 deep belly breaths or to comfort.

Relax and repeat with the left arm and right leg.

Lift just the right arm and left leg off the floor.
You can place a towel under the forehead or a pillow under the hips if needed.

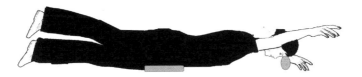

Checklist
- ✓ Press the stomach and hips into the floor and tighten the buttocks muscles to protect the back
- ✓ Lift just one arm and leg at a time. Do not lift the other arm, leg, or head off the floor
- ✓ Use a pillow under the hips &/or towel roll under the forehead if needed
- ✓ Do not lift the arm and leg too high and strain the low back
- ✓ Use diaphragmatic breathing through the nose as much as possible
- ✓ Do not exercise to the point of strain or discomfort
- ✓ Remember the goal of yoga is to find that point where you are challenging yourself but not struggling

Boat Pose

Lie on your stomach with the hands down by your sides, palms facing the floor. Place your forehead or chin on the floor. To protect the neck do not turn your head to the side. If needed, you can place a pillow under the hips (if your back is sensitive) or a towel roll under the forehead. Press your abdominal muscles and pelvic bones down into the floor and tighten the buttocks muscles. This will help to protect the back.

Begin to lift your head, shoulders, chest, legs, and arms off the floor as high as you are able. Do not tilt the head back and compress the neck. Keep your gaze down at the floor. Reach your arms back and open the chest. Make sure you do not strain the low back. Only lift as high as you can without hurting your back. Hold for 5-10 deep belly breaths or to comfort.

Lift the head, shoulders, chest, legs and arms off the floor.
You can place a towel under the forehead or a pillow under the hips if needed.

Checklist
- ✓ Press the stomach and hips into the floor and tighten the buttocks muscles to protect the back
- ✓ Do not tilt the head back and compress the neck
- ✓ Use a pillow under the hips &/or towel roll under the forehead if needed
- ✓ Do not lift the arm and leg too high and strain the low back
- ✓ Use diaphragmatic breathing through the nose as much as possible
- ✓ Do not exercise to the point of strain or discomfort
- ✓ Remember the goal of yoga is to find that point where you are challenging yourself but not struggling

Sphinx Pose

Lie on your stomach with the hands underneath your shoulders and palms facing the floor. Place your forehead or chin on the floor. If needed, you can place a pillow under the hips (if your back is sensitive) or a towel roll under the forehead. Press your abdominal muscles and pelvic bones down into the floor and tighten the buttocks muscles. This will help to protect the back.

Using your low back muscles begin to lift your head, shoulders, and chest off the floor as high as you are able. Your arms can help support you but avoid using arm strength alone to lift up. Do not tilt the head back and compress the neck. Keep your gaze down at the floor and slightly ahead. Lift as high as you can but do not strain the low back. Only lift as high as you can without hurting your back. Keep the shoulders down and away from the ears. From here, take the elbows and hands and pull back towards your body as if you were trying to slide your hips forward. This will help to lengthen through the low back versus just arching up. If coming up this high bothers your back you can rest on your elbows. Hold for 5-10 deep belly breaths or to comfort.

Full Spinx

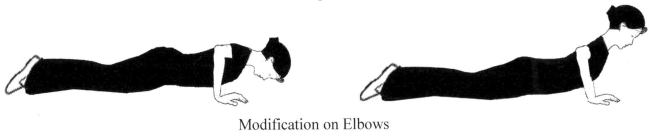

Modification on Elbows

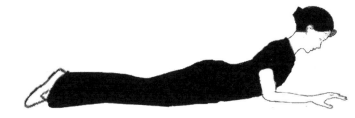

Checklist
- ✓ Press the stomach and hips into the floor and tighten the buttocks muscles to protect the back
- ✓ Do not tilt the head back and compress the neck
- ✓ Use a pillow under the hips &/or towel roll under the forehead if needed
- ✓ Use the low back muscles, not the arms to lift you up
- ✓ Do not lift high and strain the low back
- ✓ Use diaphragmatic breathing through the nose as much as possible
- ✓ Do not exercise to the point of strain or discomfort
- ✓ Remember the goal of yoga is to find that point where you are challenging yourself but not struggling

Child Pose

The last few postures have focused on arching the low back and opening the chest. It is always good to balance your practice by moving the body in opposing ways. Child pose will help to relax the low back and provides a counter stretch for the back.

Come up to hands and knees. Let the hips drop back and bring them as close to your heels as you can. Let the head relax on the floor. The object of this pose is to let your body relax. Avoid holding your head off of the floor.

If your knees are sensitive you can place a pillow between the heels and buttocks to reduce the bend in the knees. If your head will not comfortably rest on the floor place a pillow under the forehead so the neck can relax. Hold for 5-10 deep belly breaths or to comfort.

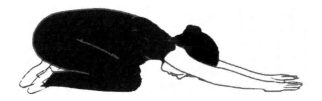

Checklist
- ✓ Use a pillow under the hips &/or forehead if needed
- ✓ To support the neck your head should be touching the floor or a pillow
- ✓ Use diaphragmatic breathing through the nose as much as possible
- ✓ Do not exercise to the point of strain or discomfort
- ✓ Remember the goal of yoga is to find that point where you are challenging yourself but not struggling

Bound Angle

The last yoga posture is a a restorative pose. The goal of this posture is to allow the body to completely relax. This posture also helps to open the shoulders and chest.

You will need a yoga bolster or you can use a couch cushion or a pile of blankets and a few pillows.

If your neck is sensitive you can use the bolster the long way so that your head stays on the bolster. If your neck does not bother you, use the bolster the short way so that your neck and head come off the end of the bolster.

To get into this posture, sit up straight and place the bolster behind you. Do not sit on the bolster. Then, lie down over the bolster. If you are using the bolster the short way have the end of the bolster come just underneath your armpits so your shoulders are off the bolster.

Place a pillow underneath each knee. The purpose of this posture is to let the whole body completely relax, so let the pillows support your knees if they do not reach the floor. The closer the heels are to the body the deeper the stretch, so adjust your heels accordingly. To support the neck you can also place a pillow or rolled up towel underneath the neck. Make sure you do not arch the neck. The head and neck should be straight. Hold this posture for as long as feels comfortable. Take deep belly breaths into the chest and shoulders and let your body sink and rest into the cushions.

Using the bolster the long way   *Using the bolster the short way*

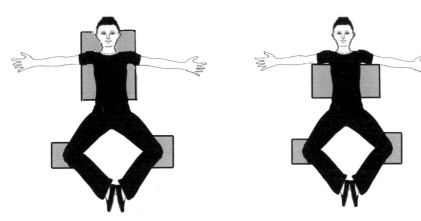

Checklist
- ✓ Make sure your neck is supported and do not let the head tip back
- ✓ Use pillows to support the knees if they do not reach the floor to allow your leg muscles to fully relax
- ✓ Use diaphragmatic breathing through the nose as much as possible
- ✓ Do not exercise to the point of strain or discomfort
- ✓ Remember the goal of yoga is to find that point where you are challenging yourself but not struggling

Chapter Five

*"If you don't like something change it; if you can't change it,
change the way you think about it"*
- Mary Engelbreit

Relaxation Techniques and Stress Management.

What is stress

Stress is not a disease but rather a normal part of everyone's life. Stress is any event that an organism must adapt to, and it does not necessarily have a negative or positive correlation. Stress results from situations that require one to change and/or adjust behaviorally and such changes can be positive or negative. Examples of stress include the body responding to the pressures of gravity, physiological adaptations to an exercise regimen, or changes to one's way of life. Stress can include feelings of mental or emotional strain, suspense, anxiety, fear, worry, tension, excitement, or a general feeling of uneasiness or dread in response to a real or imagined threat. Any sort of change can make you feel stressed, even good change. It's not just the change or event itself that matters, but how you react to it. Therefore the word stress does not always need to be associated with a negative event. What may be stressful is different for each person. For example, although one person may not feel stressed about retiring from work, another person may. Getting married is a joyous event. It is also stressful for many. Having to adjust to an illness or financial changes can be stressful. In life, we have to constantly adjust to change. Exposure to stress becomes a issue when the stressor is perceived as something to which one can not adapt to, control, or when an individual believes that he or she is unable to cope with the situation.

What happens to the body when we feel stressed

Stress is caused by the body's natural instinct to defend itself. In the case of emergencies such as getting out of the way of a speeding car this instinct is good, but it can cause physical symptoms if it goes on for too long, such as in response to life's daily challenges and changes. Stress evokes the fight-or-flight response. The fight-or-flight response is characterized by increased metabolism, heart rate, breathing, and blood pressure all of which prepare us to run or to fight, and this can lead to a number of stress-related symptoms.

In order for the above reactions to occur, the various systems of the body must signal and communicate with one another. The body-mind accomplishes this communication through the use of messenger molecules controlled by various systems of the body. These messenger molecules help to send and receive signals that activate both voluntary and involuntary actions. Some of the systems of the body include the nervous system, the neuropeptide system, the immune system, and the endocrine system.

The Nervous System

This system is comprised of the central nervous system (CNS) and the peripheral nervous system. The peripheral system connects the CNS to sensory receptors and motor neurons allowing the CNS to communicate with the muscles and glands. The peripheral nervous system is further divided into the autonomic nervous system which includes the sympathetic nervous system and the parasympathetic nervous system.

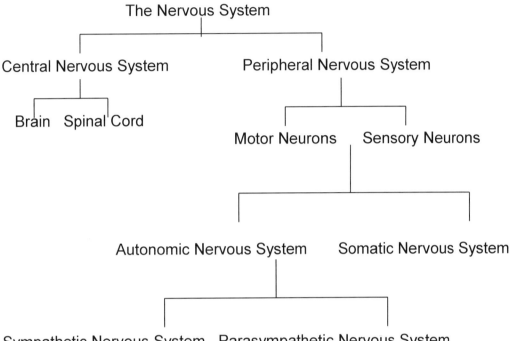

What is the stress response

Research suggests that constant exposure to even mild stress over a prolonged period of time may have a detrimental effect on the body. These studies also suggest that stress management could potentially play a role in the management and treatment of many common ailments. In cases where there is a threat to our survival or physical well being the stress response is activated as needed, but then it is deactivated when the threat has passed. However, problems occur when the stress response is not deactivated. The stress response can become a constant occurrence in our daily life - during an argument, when stuck in traffic, experiencing financial difficulties, or when facing a chronic illness. While these situations may not be life threatening, whenever the body-mind senses that you are worried or "stressed" the fight or flight response is stimulated. If you constantly feel the pressures of such situations during daily life, then your body and mind is in a constant state of arousal.

The stress response occurs when an individual is exposed to a perceived danger. Then, in less then a second, the sympathetic nervous system (SNS) is signaled to release catecholamines such as epinephrine (adrenaline) and norepinephrine (noradrenaline), that enhances rapid activation of our reflex response system. These chemicals cause an increase in heart rate, muscle tension, and blood pressure. Blood flow is diverted from the internal organs and skin, and sent to the brain and muscles. Our rate of breathing increases, our pupils dilate, and perspiration increases. The hypothalamus, interpreting the above reactions, relays information to the molecule corticotrophin-releasing hormone (CRH) as well as to other hormones. These hormones then signal the pituitary gland to release adrenocorticotrophin (ACTH) as well as other hormones in order to evoke additional adaptive responses. These adaptive responses include the release of cortisol which aids in mobilizing energy, increasing cardiovascular and cardiopulmonary activity, sharpening cognitive abilities to increase performance, and decreasing the activity of the immune and digestive systems.

After you've fought, fled or otherwise escaped your stressful situation, the parasympathetic nervous system is signaled to reverse the above process bringing the body back to a "resting" state as the levels of cortisol and adrenaline in your bloodstream decline. As a result, your heart rate and blood pressure return to normal and your digestion and metabolism resume their regular pace. This entire process involves a circular informational loop between the limbic system, hypothalamus, pituitary system, and the adrenals of the body, and back again.

The Autonomic Nervous System and the Fight Or Flight Response

Parasympathetic System	Sympathetic System
Constricts Pupil	Dilates pupil
Stimulates salivation	Inhibits salivation
Slows heartbeat	Accelerates heartbeat
Slows breathing	Accelerates breathing
Stimulates digestion	Inhibits digestion
Inhibits hormones	Activates secretion of hormones
Contracts bladder	Relaxes bladder
Relaxes rectum	Contracts rectum

What triggers the stress response

First, it is essential to understand that the body-mind does not know the difference between a real and imagined threat, for example; you are watching a frightening movie. Even though you may be sitting comfortably in your living room, and reason tells you that you are not actually in danger, your body still responds. When you see frightening images the brain interprets these as a danger or threat to the well being of the body, and in turn activates the fight or flight response. Your heart beat increases, your breathing quickens and becomes more shallow, your palms may become sweaty, and you may even physically jump or become startled. While at a much lower level this same set of reactions can occur due to a constant stream of negative thoughts or during periods of constant worry. These thoughts and worries are signals to the brain that something is wrong or that there is a threat to your well being, causing the body-mind to respond. This reaction can occur even if the thoughts we are having are merely anticipations about what might happen. Frequently our worries are about events that have not actually happened.

How does stress affect your health

As explained above, the human body is designed to experience stress and to react to it. Stress can be positive, keeping us alert and ready to avoid danger. Stress becomes negative when a person faces continual challenges without relief or relaxation between challenges. When stressful situations pile up one after another, your body has no chance to recover. As a result, one may tend to become overworked as stress-related tension builds. Stress that continues without relief can lead to physical symptoms including headaches, upset stomach, elevated blood pressure, chest pain, and problems sleeping.

The long-term activation of the stress-response system can disrupt almost all your body's processes, increasing your risk of obesity, insomnia, digestive complaints, heart disease, and depression. Research suggests that stress can also bring on or worsen certain symptoms or diseases.

Consider the following:
➤ Stress is linked to six of the leading causes of death: heart disease, cancer, lung ailments, accidents, cirrhosis of the liver, and suicide.
➤ Chronic stress can wear down the body's natural defenses and cause health problems or make problems worse if you don't learn ways to deal with it.

Stress can effect such systems of the body as:

➤ Digestive system. It's common to have a stomachache or diarrhea when you're stressed. This happens because stress hormones slow the release of stomach acid and the emptying of the stomach. The same hormones also stimulate the colon, which speeds the passage of its contents. Chronic stress can also lead to continuously high levels of cortisol. This hormone can increase appetite and cause weight gain.

➤ Immune system. Chronic stress tends to decrease the activity of your immune system, making you more susceptible to colds and other infections. Normally, your immune system responds to infection by releasing several substances that cause inflammation. In response, the adrenal glands produce cortisol, which switches off the immune and inflammatory responses once the infection is cleared. However, prolonged stress keeps your cortisol levels continuously elevated, so your immune system remains suppressed.

In some cases, stress can have the opposite effect, making your immune system overactive. The result is an increased risk of autoimmune diseases where your immune system attacks your body's own cells. Stress can also worsen the symptoms of autoimmune diseases.

➢ Nervous system. If your fight-or-flight response never shuts off, stress hormones produce persistent feelings of anxiety, helplessness and impending doom. Oversensitivity to stress has been linked with severe depression, possibly because depressed people have a harder time adapting to the negative effects of cortisol. The byproducts of cortisol act as sedatives, which contribute to the overall feeling of depression. Excessive amounts of cortisol can cause sleep disturbances, a lessening of the sex drive and loss of appetite.

➢ Cardiovascular system. High levels of cortisol can also raise your heart rate and increase your blood pressure and blood lipid (cholesterol and triglyceride) levels. These are risk factors for both heart attacks and strokes. Cortisol levels also appear to play a role in the accumulation of abdominal fat, which gives some people an "apple" shape. People with apple body shapes have a higher risk of heart disease and diabetes than do people with "pear" body shapes, where weight is more concentrated in the hips.

➢ Other systems. Stress may worsen such skin conditions as psoriasis, eczema, hives and acne, and it can be a trigger for asthma attacks.

Signs and symptoms of stress

Physical	Behavioral	Emotional
Headaches	Restlessness	Crying
Indigestion	Being overly critical of others	Nervousness
Stomach aches	Grinding one's teeth at night	Anxiety
Sweaty palms	Inability to get things done or make decisions	Boredom (there's no meaning to anything)
Hypertension (high blood pressure)	Easily upset	Edginess (a readiness to explode)
Dizziness or a general feeling of "being out of it"	Excessive anger and hostility	Feeling powerless to change things
Tension in the back, neck, face, and shoulders	Lack of creativity	An overwhelming sense of pressure
Heart irregularities	Problems with relationships	Loneliness
Insomnia	Loss of interest in activities	Depression
Tiredness	Withdrawing from relationships	Constant worry
Trembling/shaking		Loss of sense of humor
Constipation or diarrhea		
Shortness of breath		

Stress and MS

The prolonged stress of living with a condition such as MS can lead to frustration, anger, hopelessness, and depression. There are often worries about:
- Uncertainty about having MS/waiting for a correct diagnosis
- The unpredictability of the course of the disease
- Symptoms that are invisible to others
- The need to adjust as symptoms change or emerge
- Financial and work concerns
- Loss of control of muscle function
- Starting and modifying the many prescription drugs used to manage the condition

Stress management is essential in the effective management of MS because some symptoms of MS can get worse under stress. Therefore, the right amount of rest along with a regular program of stress management is a very important part of controlling the symptoms of MS.

Techniques to reduce and manage stress
➢ Learn to recognize when you're feeling stressed and become conscious of your reaction to the stress.
➢ Choose a way to deal with your stress.
  If possible avoid the event or situation that leads to your stress. Identify areas of your life you can change to eliminate or reduce exposure to stress.
  To the best of your ability prepare for events you know may be stressful (a job interview or doctor's appointment).
  Do any unpleasant tasks first thing in the morning so you will not worry about it all day.
➢ If you can not avoid the situation, change how you react to stress.
  Try to look at change as a positive challenge, not a threat. Step back from the conflict or worry and shift your outlook. Many times, simply choosing to look at situations in a more positive way can reduce the amount of stress in your life.
➢ Don't worry about things you can't control (the weather or others actions).
➢ Teach yourself to control your physical reactions to stress.
➢ Build up your emotional ability to deal with stress.
➢ Simplify things and relax your standards. It is Ok if the dishes do not get done right away or let go of needing everything to be done perfectly.
➢ If the morning rush is stressful commit to getting up a bit earlier, do some of the preparation the night before, make sure that all of your morning tasks are absolutely necessary.
➢ Do one thing at a time. Let yourself completely finish one task before worrying about or starting the next. Having too many projects going at one time is stressful.
➢ Learn to say no to things you really do not have the time or energy for.
➢ Ask for help from friends, family or professionals.

Take a break, talk to someone close and get a different perspective on your troubles. Work to resolve conflicts with other people. On your own, you may have limited success trying to change the habitual patterns of thought and behavior that trigger your stress response. Psychiatrists, psychologists, and licensed clinical social workers are trained to help you break free of these patterns. The most important step you can take is to seek help as soon as you feel less able to cope. Taking action early will enable you to understand and deal with the many effects of MS.

➤ Set realistic goals at home and at work.
➤ Exercise on a regular basis. Exercise increases your physical capacity to deal with stress
➤ Eat well-balanced meals and get enough sleep.
➤ Get away from your daily stresses by participating in group sports, social events, and hobbies.
➤ Remember, it is not your fault that you have MS. There is *no guilt* attached to having MS. You must believe this - consciously and subconsciously!
➤ Take control. Exercise, join a support group, look outside yourself, help others. Talking with others in an MS support group helps you connect with people who understand what you are coping with.
 Find out as much as you can about the illness.
 Talk to your friends and family about it. Do not isolate them. They will want to be involved in helping you.
➤ Do something you enjoy every day.
➤ Meditate or practice relaxation techniques.

Stress management requires continuous practice as you go through life and deal with change — which often comes unexpectedly. Even if you take everyday frustrations in stride, your stress response can still surge up when you find yourself dealing with something big, such as illness, job loss, or bereavement.

MS and depression

Some of the symptoms of stress are very similar to those of depression and can mimic the symptoms of MS. A common sign of depression is the loss of interest in activities you once enjoyed. If you think that you or someone you know is depressed or if there are five or more of the following symptoms that continue for two or more weeks without improvement you may want to talk with your doctor or healthcare provider.

- Sleeping too much or too little.
- Marked changes in appetite or weight loss or gain.
- Agitation and anxiety.
- Decreased energy and increased fatigue.
- Feelings of worthlessness, guilt, or self doubt.
- Memory loss, difficulty concentrating or making decisions.

- Feeling sad or down in the dumps most of the day, nearly every day.
- Loss of interest in activities that you once looked forward to.
- Thoughts of death, suicide or harming yourself.

How practicing meditation and relaxation techniques can help manage stress

Meditation and relaxation techniques are forms of focused concentration that work by introducing calm, peaceful images in the mind, creating a "mental escape." Meditation techniques provide a powerful psychological strategy that enhances a person's coping skills. Many people dealing with stress feel a loss of control, fear, panic, anxiety, helplessness, and uncertainty. Research has shown that practicing meditation and relaxation techniques can help people overcome stress, anger, pain, depression, insomnia, and other problems associated with illnesses and medical/surgical procedures. Stress and depression can worsen the symptoms of MS. Meditation and relaxation techniques help you to remain calm. In addition to reducing stress and depression, meditation and relaxation techniques can:

➢ Dramatically decrease pain and the need for pain medication
➢ Decrease side effects and complications of medical procedures
➢ Shorten hospital stays and reduce recovery time
➢ Enhance sleep
➢ Strengthen the immune system and enhance the ability to heal
➢ Increase self-confidence and self-control

Meditation/Relaxation Techniques

There are many types of meditation or relaxation techniques. All aim for the same outcome they simply utilize different techniques. Experiment with the different techniques in order to find one that works well for you. You may also find that some techniques work best in certain circumstances.

Basic meditation/relaxation
When practicing this basic technique the physiological and psychological reactions that occur in the body are the exact opposite of those which happen during the activation of the fight or flight response. By regularly eliciting this calmer state, one may be able to counteract the detrimental effects of constant stress. When the fight or flight response is activated several reactions occur. These include an increase in heart rate, blood pressure, rate of respiration, muscular tension, and blood flow being directed away from the process of digestion and instead directed towards the muscles and brain. When the basic meditation exercise is practiced the exact opposite can occur. There may be a reduction in heart rate, rate of respiration, muscular tension, and an overall decrease in the body's metabolism.

Basic meditation technique

The goal of the basic meditation exercise is to allow the mind to shift away from the constant stream of thoughts and worries and instead focus solely on the movement of the breath. This helps to slow down the activity and chatter in the mind, which in turn will send signals to the body-mind that you are relaxed and there is nothing to worry about. As the body-mind receives these calming signals, the brain will signal the body to calm the nervous system and reverse the effects of the fight or flight syndrome. You may also find that after meditating you may be less likely to rush around and more inclined to remain in the peaceful state you achieved during your relaxation session.

Basic Meditation Steps

1) Find a quiet place where you will not be disturbed for about 15-20 minutes. Turn off phones and remove as many distractions as possible.

2) Find a comfortable position that you can remain in for about 15-20 minutes. This can be sitting in a chair with the back straight but not rigid and feet flat on the floor, or sitting cross-legged on the floor. If you find sitting cross-legged on the floor uncomfortable on your knees or back, you can sit on a cushion or pillow in order to raise your hips a bit higher then your knees. This will help to both take pressure off of the knees and maintain a straight back. You can also lie down for this exercise, as long as you do not fall asleep.

3) Close the eyes and begin to focus on your breath.
Inhale through the nose and allow your abdominal area to rise, as if you were filling this area with air. Exhale through the nose and allow the stomach to fall as the air leaves this area. Sometimes it is easier to start with the exhalation and just once, contract the abdominal muscles and push the air out. Then allow the stomach to relax and rise with the inhalation. It is normal for this style of breathing to feel backwards or awkward at first but with practice it will become easier.

For the next 20 minutes remain focused on your breath. To keep the mind focused allow yourself to be aware of the abdomen as it rises and falls, or allow your attention to remain on the sensation of the air as it enters and exits the nose. If these sensations are difficult to focus on, the breath can be counted by silently saying one on the inhale and two on the exhale. If the mind does wander, which it will, simply without judgement bring your attention back to the breath.

When first attempting this exercise you may need to bring your attention back quite often. However, keeping your attention on the breath and away from other thoughts will become easier with practice. You can time yourself for the 20 minutes, however, avoid using a loud alarm as you do not want to startle the body out of meditation. An alarm which can be programmed to come on with soft music could be used. It is not recommended to continually open the eyes and look at the time as this disrupts the process of concentrated meditation. You can also play very soft music for 20 minutes as a way to time yourself. When the 20 minutes is up, allow yourself time and do not get up too quickly. Take a few minutes to feel the results of your meditation.

4) Remember to keep a passive attitude. Meditation is a skill and like any new skill, takes practice. Remember to not get concerned about doing the exercise correctly and be careful about expecting any particular results. The object is to simply take time out of the day to give the body-mind a break from everyday thoughts and worries.

Note:

The breathing is taught in and out of the nose, since this is physiologically more relaxing for the body. However if you are experiencing respiratory or sinus issues and find this difficult you can breathe through the mouth. You may find that with practice, breathing strictly through the nose will become easier.

Autogenic Training (AT)

This technique trains the body-mind to become quiet and relaxed by utilizing self-suggestions. These self-suggestions attempt to change the thoughts present in the mind, by suggesting to the body-mind that certain events are occurring. These events can include a slower heartbeat, increased blood flow, and less muscle tension. Since research suggests the possibility that negative thoughts can result in decreased efficiency of the systems in the body, advocates of AT suggest that we can utilize positive thoughts to enhance the efficiency of the systems of the body.

Autogenic Training exercise

If you find that these particular suggestions do not apply to your situation, please feel free to substitute any other "suggestions." You may wish to record these instructions onto a tape until you are more familiar with the process.

Find a comfortable position which you can remain in for about 20 minutes where you will not be disturbed. Begin to focus on your breath and allow your body to relax. Slowly and silently count down from four to one. When you reach the number 1 you will be completely relaxed.

Concentrate on your right arm. Slowly and silently say to yourself six times, my right arm is very heavy.

Concentrate on your left arm. Slowly and silently say to yourself six times, my left arm is very heavy.

Concentrate on both arms. Slowly and silently say to yourself six times, my arms are very heavy.

Turn your attention away from your arms, and silently say to yourself just once, I am very quiet, and I enjoy feeling relaxed for a while.

Concentrate on your right leg. Slowly and silently say to yourself six times, my right leg is very heavy.

Concentrate on your left leg. Slowly and silently say to yourself six times my left leg is very heavy.

Concentrate on both legs. Slowly and silently say to yourself six times my legs are very heavy.

Turn your attention away from your legs, and silently say to yourself just once, I am very quiet, and I enjoy feeling relaxed for a while.

Concentrate on the beating of your heart. Slowly and silently say to yourself six times, my heartbeat is calm and strong.

Turn your attention away from your heartbeat, and silently say to yourself just once, I am very quiet and I enjoy feeling relaxed for a while.

Concentrate on the rhythm of your breathing. Slowly and silently say to yourself six times, my breathing is slow and deep.

Turn your attention away from your breath and silently say to yourself just once, I am very quiet and I enjoy feeling relaxed for a while.

Concentrate on your stomach. Slowly and silently say to yourself six times, warmth is radiating throughout my stomach and throughout my body.

Turn your attention away from your stomach and silently say to yourself just once, I am very quiet and I enjoy feeling relaxed, for a while.

Concentrate on your forehead. Slowly and silently say to yourself six times, my forehead is cool.

Turn your attention away from your forehead and silently say to yourself just once, I am very quiet and I enjoy feeling relaxed, for a while.

Bring your attention back to your breath.
Slowly and silently count down from four to one. By the time you reach the number one, you will be alert and awake, yet relaxed.

Begin to circle the wrists and ankles, gently stretching and moving the body. When you are ready, slowly open the eyes. Take a few minutes to feel the effects of your meditation.

Guided Imagery

Where Autogenic Training utilizes self-suggestion, guided imagery relies on images to suggest physiological changes to the body-mind creating harmony between the mind and body. Guided imagery or visualization is a process by which you create calm, peaceful images in your mind in order to help elicit a state of relaxation or manage symptoms.

Guided imagery, much like the basic meditation exercise, aims to present the brain with different stimuli to focus on, allowing for a break from everyday thoughts and worries. Imagery is often used to stimulate changes in bodily functions that are usually considered inaccessible to conscious influence. Imagery can be effective, as research suggests that the brain will respond to mentally created images much in the same way it responds to actually seeing images. A common example of how this works is to try the following exercise.

First try to imagine a lemon… Use all of your senses… Smell the lemon and get a sense of its texture… Next, recall what a lemon tastes like… Now imagine cutting open the lemon and squirting some of the lemon juice into your mouth… Imagine swishing the lemon juice around in your mouth and then swallowing it.

In this exercise even though tasting the lemon was only in your imagination you may have noticed changes in your body. You might have begun to salivate and you might have even puckered at the thought of the taste. In this example your body-mind responded to the thought as though the event actually took place. Constant worry is another example of the effects of imagery. As you worry about events that may or may not happen, your body-mind may respond by tensing muscles and arousing the nervous system in anticipation of a challenge.

Imagery can also provide a way to communicate conscious intentions or requests to your unconscious mind. When using guided imagery the participant might visualize a scene such as a beach, meadow, or other such place which can elicit feelings of relaxation and peace. In this example when imagining such a scene, the body-mind receives signals that it is all right to relax since there is no threat present. Imagery may also be used when dealing with a particular disease such as cancer. In this case the patient may use imagery to visualize the body-mind healing itself from the disease by "seeing" or imagining their immune system eliminating the cancerous cells. Imagery, like many of the complementary techniques available can be used in conjunction with medical treatment.

For someone who is taking medication for an illness, imagery could be used to visualize the treatment working. As with most all forms of meditation, the practice of guided imagery or visualization can help to interrupt the flow of constant thoughts and worries, and thereby allow the body-mind to rest, conserve energy, and build energy reserves.

Using guided imagery (or other types of meditation) to manage stress and symptoms can provide a sense of hope and encourage feelings of control over one's situation. However, as with any form of meditation, a passive attitude is essential. While it is important to make the images as real as possible, it is just as important to not focus on results or particular outcomes. When an end result or outcome is the focus, anxiety and tension can result which are counterproductive to stress and symptom management.

When first practicing guided imagery it may seem difficult to actually "see" the images. It is important to know that with practice, visualizing images will become easier. It is important to not become frustrated or tense if visualization exercises do not come easily. Sometimes it may be easier to "sense" the image versus struggling to "see" the image. For example if trying to visualize a healing light, instead of "seeing" the light you may choose to just "sense" that it is there, by focusing on a sensation of warmth or heat, a tingling sensation, or just simply knowing that it is there.

In order to practice guided imagery you can try some simple exercises. First notice a basic object around your home. Make it something simple without a lot of design. Observe the object for a few minutes and really notice its detail. Then, close your eyes and try to recall the object in your mind's eye. Try this with various objects keeping it simple at first, and then work up to more detailed objects.

Guided Imagery/Visualization Exercise.

There are many different versions of imagery exercises, however the example below is a commonly used technique. It will be easier to either record the instructions on a tape or have someone read them to you so you can remain focused on the process versus continually having to stop and look at the directions. As with the basic meditation exercise, find a way to time yourself so you are not startled out of the meditation. You will need approximately twenty minutes for this exercise.

1) Begin by practicing the basic meditation technique for approximately five to ten minutes. The time does not need to be exact, but it should be long enough for you to feel a shift in the state of tension and relaxation of your body.
The following is the script to use for the imagery section. Where I have included "….." signals a time to give yourself a few minutes in-between the next instruction.

2) Begin to imagine yourself walking on a private beach on a perfect summer day………
Take some time to look around and use all of your senses to explore the area………
Hear the waves as they come up gently on the shore……….
Feel the warm sun on your skin and the sand underneath your feet…………
Smell the salt air……….. notice how being here makes you feel……………

Find a place where you can sit or lie down either on the shore, in the water, or anywhere else that looks inviting to you…………..
Begin to become aware of the light and warmth from the sun…………
As you relax here allow this warmth and light to permeate your skin and be absorbed into the body………
Allow yourself to imagine this light and warmth to have healing properties………….
If there are any areas of tightness, tension, or disease present in the body-mind allow these things to be dissolved by the warmth and light…………….
Take some time here to relax and heal the body-mind……………
(allow 10-15 min. here for this experience)

Begin to bring your attention back to the breath…………….
Feel the abdomen rise as you inhale and the abdomen fall as you exhale……..
Allow yourself to slowly and gently become a little more awake and a little more alert with each breath…………..become aware of the pressures against your body from the floor or chair………..
Then when you are ready slowly open the eyes.

3) Allow yourself to come out of the meditation slowly and take some time to feel the effects of the exercise.

4) Remember to maintain a passive attitude. Visualizing images can be difficult at first, however, it will become easier with practice. If you find visualizing the above difficult, you can try to focus on sensation instead. In this example, you would allow yourself to feel the sensation of being at a relaxed spot, and focus more on the sensation of the warmth of the sun entering your body versus focusing on actually visualizing the light.

Mindfulness Meditation

This form of meditation, which has its roots in Buddhism, is focused on learning to become fully present in the moment and to be fully accepting of whatever is occurring in the present moment. Unlike the three other forms of meditation presented, this form of meditation aims to help the participant change their response to stimuli rather then alter their physiology. The goal is for the meditator to be fully aware of the stimuli around them, (such as noise or other people), yet learn to not react to the stimuli. This process is also referred to as learning to become a dispassionate watcher or a witness. During this process the participant aims to become aware of the mind's constant stream of thoughts and to it's constant judgement and reaction to inner and outer experiences. This technique aims to teach one how to not get caught up in these thoughts by allowing oneself to step back from the thoughts.

An example of this would be meditating while experiencing pain. In the basic meditation exercise, the participant tries to interrupt the pain signals, and the typical anxiety laden thoughts that accompany them, by shifting the mind's attention onto awareness of the breath, since interrupting the flow of thoughts can often aid in reducing symptoms. Autogenic Training would utilize self-suggestions such as the area which is painful, is becoming more relaxed and is therefore more comfortable. In the case of guided imagery the participant might try mentally visualizing the pain as a red ball which then turns into a softer color and becomes smaller and smaller until the ball disappears. With these types of meditation the aim is to interrupt the stream of thoughts which are occurring in the mind, but also suggest to the body-mind that the pain no longer exists.

However, when using mindfulness meditation, the participant would not attempt any of the above. Rather the meditator would acknowledge the pain but attempt to not react to it with thoughts of anger, depression or frustration. Approaching the sensation of pain in this way gives the body-mind an alternate way of seeing discomfort. Instead of becoming agitated by the sensation the meditator would relate to the experience or sensation of pain simply as an event that is happening in the present, but would refrain from allowing the mind to wander to negative thoughts about the sensation. In other words the meditator would not allow the mind to become distracted with thoughts which attempt to predict what the pain may or may not do in the future, or how the pain effects their life. This process attempts to run interference so that thoughts, emotions and/or memories do not integrate the experience of pain with the activation of the fight or flight response. This form of meditation can help the participant to learn to lessen the times the body-mind is activated when exposed to stress.

The limbic system (the emotional center of the brain) is directly linked to the hypothalamus region which aids in the regulation of the autonomic nervous system. By learning to not allow emotions to take charge (getting angry about the pain) the hypothalamus in turn does not receive the signal to activate the stress response. This form of meditation is based on a fundamental Buddhist belief - that the origin of much of our suffering comes from a constant need to grasp onto things and the attempt to change what is.

Mindfulness Meditation Exercise

Below is a sample of a typical mindfulness meditation exercise. As with the other forms of meditation, find a way to time yourself for twenty minutes so you will not be startled out of the exercise.

1) Begin by practicing the basic meditation technique for approximately five to ten minutes. The time does not need to be exact, but it should be long enough for you to feel a shift in the state of tension and relaxation of your body.

2) When your body-mind has quieted down, try shifting your awareness to the process of thinking and take your attention off of the breath. Attempt to be a dispassionate observer as you simply "watch" the thoughts that come into your mind. Try to perceive the thoughts simply as events in your mind. Try to not allow yourself to

become caught up in the thoughts, just notice that they are there. Notice their content and the rate at which they change. Notice that each particular thought does not last very long, but rather individual thoughts come and go, and sometimes the same thought will keep coming back. If you notice sensations of discomfort, allow yourself to become aware of the sensations, yet choose to not react to them. Notice if the sensations change with time. Again try to practice being the observer of an event. Notice if by simply observing the sensation you can allow yourself to become detached from the sensation. (However if you are experiencing significant discomfort do not force yourself to continue with this exercise).

To end the meditation bring your awareness back to your breathing for a few minutes.

3) End the meditation slowly and allow yourself a few minutes to experience the effects of this exercise.

4) Remember to maintain a passive attitude. Try to avoid getting caught up in how well you performed the meditation or becoming attached to any particular results.

This form of meditation can be challenging at first. You may find it difficult to stay with this exercise for a full 20 minutes. If this occurs, start by practicing for just a few minutes at a time and slowly build up to a 15-20 minute practice.

Resource Section

This book has covered many techniques and forms of movement, which can help in managing the symptoms and challenges faced by those with MS. In addition there are many other opinions, approaches, and techniques not covered in this book. We encourage you to explore all of the options available and try many different approaches. With exploration you will find the approach that works best for your unique situation.

This section will provide sample routines, workout logs, and suggestions for using the information in this book. These are provided as a guide only to help you in getting started in developing your own routine. As you learn how different movements affect you, you can then work to develop your own routine. The following are general suggestions concerning the use of movement therapy for those with MS.

For the best results, you need to do some exercise everyday. You do not need to do all of the exercises in this book every day. It is best to alter your routine between a variety of exercises. Doing the same exact workout every time you exercise will cause the body to adapt to the routine and lessen the affect of the exercise. To keep the body responding to exercise it is important to periodically change your routine or change the amount or type of resistance you are using.

The following list provides information on the exercises that are important to do everyday and exercises which are best if done two or three times per week

➢ Things you should try to do everyday include:
   1. Deep diaphragmatic breathing exercises. Try for 10-15 minutes of deep breathing each day.
   2. Stretching to relax the muscles and maintain joint range of motion.
   3. Balancing exercises.
   4. Relaxation technique.

➢ Things you should do at least two to three times per week.
   1. Aerobic or cardiovascular exercise. This can either be the aerobic exercises from chapter two or walking. During the week you can alternate the aerobic exercises with a brisk 15-30 minute walk. You should walk at a pace that gets your heart rate up and you should feel slightly out of breath. Make sure you use correct walking form (pg. 25) using heel-toe walking and swing your arms (opposite arm to leg). An indicator of good cardiovascular health is being able to complete a 15-minute mile. This may be too fast of a pace, but gives you something to aim for.
   2. Strengthening exercises for the arms, legs, and abdominal muscles.
   3. A full body stretching routine.

At least once per week, get down on the floor and practice getting back up (pg. 35). Keep yourself in practice of getting up and down off of the floor. Then if you should fall you will know how to get up without having to wait for assistance.

Sample Weekly Routine 1

You do not need to do the exercises all at the same time, they can be done throughout the day. Remember, the following routines are "the ideal" involving some exercise every day. There may be times when you miss your workout or are not feeling up to exercise, or are only able to do part of it. Use your own judgement as to what is best for your body, and how much exercise is appropriate. Make a commitment to exercise as often as you realistically can and be gentle with your body when needed. These routines take approximately one hour per day.

Monday
Aerobic exercises.
Strength training exercises.
10-15 minutes of deep breathing and meditation technique.

Tuesday
Walk for 15-20 minutes or to tolerance.
Yoga exercises.
10-15 minutes of deep breathing and meditation technique.

Wednesday
Aerobic exercises.
Strength training exercises.
10-15 minutes of deep breathing and meditation technique.

Thursday
Walk for 15-20 minutes or to tolerance.
Yoga exercises.
10-15 minutes of deep breathing and meditation technique.

Friday
Aerobic exercises.
Strength training exercises.
10-15 minutes of deep breathing and meditation technique.

Saturday
Some type of aerobic exercise different from walking or the aerobic exercises in this book. Examples include swimming, water walking, or some sport you enjoy.
10-15 minutes of deep breathing and meditation technique.

Sunday
Pick an activity you enjoy to get the body moving and challenge your balance.
10-15 minutes of deep breathing and meditation technique.

Sample Weekly Routine 2

Monday
Aerobic exercises.
Upper body strength training exercises.
Light stretching
10-15 minutes of deep breathing and meditation technique.

Tuesday
Walk for 15-20 minutes or to tolerance.
Lower body strength training exercises.
Yoga exercises.
10-15 minutes of deep breathing and meditation technique.

Wednesday
Aerobic exercises.
Upper body strength training exercises.
Light stretching.
10-15 minutes of deep breathing and meditation technique.

Thursday
Walk for 15-20 minutes or to tolerance.
Lower body strength training exercises.
Yoga exercises.
10-15 minutes of deep breathing and meditation technique.

Friday
Aerobic exercises.
Upper body strength training exercises.
Light stretching.
10-15 minutes of deep breathing and meditation technique.

Saturday
Some type of aerobic exercise different from walking or the aerobic exercises in this book. Examples include swimming, water walking, or some sport you enjoy.
10-15 minutes of deep breathing and meditation technique.

Sunday
Pick an activity you enjoy to get the body moving and challenge your balance.
10-15 minutes of deep breathing and meditation technique.

Workout Logs

You can use these logs to keep track of your progress for the aerobic and strength training exercises. Keeping a record of your workouts helps you to stay on track and can help motivate you to continue as you see the increase in your exercise tolerance.

In the boxes mark down the amount of time you competed each exercise. There are blank boxes provided to write in your own activities.

SAMPLE
Aerobic exercise log

Week of _01___ /_ 05___ /_04___

Warm up first

	Sun.	Mon.	Tues.	Wed.	Thurs.	Fri.	Sat.
March in place		1 min.		2 min.		1 min.	
Straight leg kick		1 min.		2 min.		1 min.	
Step side to side		1 min.		2 min.		1 min.	
Knee lifts		1 min.		2 min.		1 min.	
Side toe taps or jumping jacks		1 min.		2 min.		1 min.	
Heel taps		1 min.		2 min.		1 min.	
Walking			20 min.		15 min.		20 min.
Swimming	20 min.						

Aerobic exercise log

Week of ____/____/____

Warm up first

	Sun.	Mon.	Tues.	Wed.	Thurs.	Fri.	Sat.
March in place							
Straight leg kick							
Step side to side							
Knee lifts							
Side toe taps or jumping jacks							
Heel taps							
Walking							
Swimming							

Use this log to record the amount of weight you use and the number of repetitions you complete.

SAMPLE
Strength training log
Week of __01__ / __05__ / __04__

	Sun.	Mon.	Tues.	Wed.	Thurs.	Fri.	Sat.
Leg extension		10 reps 3 pounds		10 reps 3 pounds		10 reps 3 pounds	
Wall Slides		10 reps		10 reps		10 reps	
Side leg lift		10 reps 3 pounds		10 reps 3 pounds		10 reps 3 pounds	
Leg lift back/ Heel curl		10 reps 3 pounds		10 reps 3 pounds		10 reps 3 pounds	
Leg crossover		10 reps 3 pounds		10 reps 3 pounds		10 reps 3 pounds	
Heel raises		10 reps 3 pounds		10 reps 3 pounds		10 reps 3 pounds	
Toe Raises		10 reps 3 pounds		10 reps 3 pounds		10 reps 3 pounds	
Wall pushups or chest fly			12 reps		12 reps		12 reps
Bent row			10 reps 2 pounds		10 reps 2 pounds		10 reps 2 pounds
Front lateral raise			10 reps 2 pounds		10 reps 2 pounds		10 reps 2 pounds
Military press			10 reps 2 pounds		10 reps 2 pounds		10 reps 2 pounds
Deltoid raise			10 reps 2 pounds		10 reps 2 pounds		10 reps 2 pounds
Biceps curl			10 reps 2 pounds		10 reps 2 pounds		10 reps 2 pounds
Triceps kickback			10 reps 2 pounds		10 reps 2 pounds		10 reps 2 pounds
Wrist curls			10 reps 2 pounds		10 reps 2 pounds		10 reps 2 pounds
Reverse wrist curls			10 reps 2 pounds		10 reps 2 pounds		10 reps 2 pounds
Lean backs or bicycles		12 reps		12 reps		12 reps	
Side bends		10 reps 2 pounds		10 reps 2 pounds		10 reps 2 pounds	
Pelvic Tilt		10 reps		10 reps		10 reps	
Knee to chest		10 reps		10 reps		10 reps	
Bridge		10 reps		10 reps		10 reps	
Supine leg lift		10 reps		10 reps		10 reps	

179

Strength training log

Week of ____/____/____

	Sun.	Mon.	Tues.	Wed.	Thurs.	Fri.	Sat.
Leg extension							
Wall slides							
Side leg lift							
Leg lift back/ Heel curl							
Leg crossover							
Heel raises							
Toe Raises							
Wall pushups or chest fly							
Bent row							
Front lateral raise							
Military press							
Deltoid raise							
Biceps curl							
Triceps kickback							
Wrist curls							
Reverse wrist curls							
Lean backs or bicycles							
Side bends							
Pelvic Tilt							
Knee to chest							
Bridge							
Supine leg lift							

Yoga Log

Week of ____/____/____

List the number of repetitions done and/or how long you held each stretch for

	Sun	Mon	Tues	Wed	Thurs	Fri	Sat
Neck Rolls & stretch							
Head rotation & stretch							
Shoulder rolls							
Seated spinal twist & stretch							
Chest opener							
Chest stretch							
Arm circles							
Overhead stretch							
Toe & heel lifts							
Ankle circles							
Mountain pose							
Warrior one							
Warrior two							
Lateral angle							
Warrior three							
Tree pose							
Dancers pose							
Knee to chest							
Hamstring stretch							
Inner thigh stretch							
Outer hip stretch							
Spinal twist							
Prone arm lift							
Prone leg lift							
Half boat							
Boat pose							
Spinx pose							
Child pose							
Bound angle							

Diary for Stress Management/Meditation Exercises

Many of our clients have found it helpful to keep diaries or journals as part of their stress management program. Below is a sample page we use in our program. You can use one sheet for each time you practice or you may wish to write in a diary or journal.

.

Technique Used _____

Time of day you practiced _____

Length of time you practiced _____

How did you feel before your practice?

_____

_____

How did you feel after your practice?

_____

_____

List any experiences which you decided to respond to differently than you usually would.

_____

_____

Helpful Organizations and Webpages

Information on MS (Treatment, education, research and services)

The National Multiple Sclerosis Society
733 Third Avenue
New York, NY 10017
Phone: (800) 344-4867
www.nmss.org

Multiple Sclerosis Association of America
706 Haddonfield Road
Cherry Hill, NJ 08002
Phone: (800) 532-7667
www.msaa.com

Multiple Sclerosis Foundation, Inc.
6350 North Andrews Avenue
Fort Lauderdale, FL 33309
Phone: (800) 441-7055
www.msfacts.org

Consortium of MS Centers
c/o Gimbel MS Center
718 Teaneck RD
Teaneck, NJ 07666
Phone: (201) 837-0727
www.mscare.org

NIH Neurological Institute
P.O. Box 5801
Bethesda, MD 20824
Phone: (800) 352-9424
www.ninds.nih.gov

U.S. National Library of Medicine
8600 Rockville Pike
Bethesda, MD 20894
www.nlm.nih.gov/medlineplus/multiplesclerosis.html

Nutrition Information
American Dietetic Association Headquarters
120 South Riverside Plaza, Suite 2000
Chicago, IL 60606-6995
Phone: (800) 877-1600
www.eatright.org/Public

Food and Drug Administration
5600 Fishers Lane
Rockville, Maryland 20857
Phone: (888) 463-6332

Information on fitness (Exercise, healthy lifestyle topics, finding a qualified instructor)

American College Of Sports Medicine
P.O. Box 1440
Indianapolis, IN 46206-1440
Phone: (317) 637-9200
www.acsm.org

National Institute of Health
9000 Rockville Pike
Bethesda, Maryland 20892
Phone: (301) 496-4000
www.nih.gov

All about Multiple Sclerosis
www.mult-sclerosis.org

Information on yoga (Types of yoga, postures, books, videos, tapes, finding a qualified instructor)

Kripalu Center for Yoga and Health
P.O. Box 793
West Street, Route 183
Lenox, MA 01240
Phone: (800) 741-7353
www.kripalu.org

National Yoga Alliance
7801 Old Branch Avenue Suite 400
Clinton, MD 20735
Phone: (877) 964-2255
www.nationalyogaalliance.org

Yoga Journal
475 Sansome Street, Suite 850
San Francisco, CA 94111
Phone: (415) 591-0555,
www.yogajournal.com

Information on stress management and meditation (Forms of meditation, techniques, videos, tape

Academy for Guided Imagery
30765 Pacific Coast Highway, Suite 369
Malibu, CA 90265
Phone: (800) 726-2070
www.academyforguidedimagery.com

Bernie Siegel/ECAP
522 Jackson Park Drive
Meadville, PA 16335
Phone: (814) 337-8192
www.ecap-online.org

Jon Kabat-Zin
Stress Reduction Tapes
P.O. Box 547
Lexington, MA 02420
www.mindfulnesstapes.com

The Mind Body Medical Institute at Beth Israel Deaconess Hospital
824 Boylston Street
Chestnut Hill, MA 02467
Phone: (617) 991-0102
www.mbmi.com

Thich Nhat Hahn
Plum Village
www.plumvillage.org

Umass Medical Center
The Center for Mindfulness in Medicine, Health Care, and Society
55 Lake Avenue North Worcester, MA 01655
Phone: (508) 856-2656
www.umassmed.edu/cfm

Information on physical therapy (How physical therapy can help, health articles finding a therapist)
American Physical Therapy Association
1111 North Fairfax Street
Alexandria, VA 22314-1488
Phone: (800) 999-2782
www.apta.org

It is often helpful to check your local library for further resources.

Index

70321396R00104

Made in the USA
Columbia, SC
04 May 2017